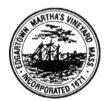

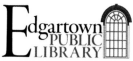

The Salt Fix

TITLE

Comments

Please share your thoughts about this book with the next borrower. Thank you!

_____

_____

_____

_____

_____

_____

_____

_____

How do you rate this book?

EXCELLENT	GOOD	FAIR	POOR

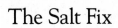

The Salt Fix

The Salt Fix

Why the Experts Got It

All Wrong—and How Eating More

Might Save Your Life

Dr. James DiNicolantonio

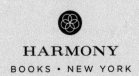

HARMONY

BOOKS · NEW YORK

Library of Congress Cataloging-in-Publication Data
Names: DiNicolantonio, James, author.
Title: The salt fix : why the experts got it all wrong—and how eating
more might save your life / Dr. James DiNicolantonio.
Description: New York : Harmony, 2017. | Includes bibliographical
references and index.
Identifiers: LCCN 2016053071 | ISBN 9780451496966 (hardback)
Subjects: LCSH: Minerals in human nutrition. | Salt. | BISAC:
MEDICAL / Nutrition. | HEALTH & FITNESS / Nutrition. |
MEDICAL / Research.
Classification: LCC QP533 .D54 2017 | DDC 613.2/8522—dc23
LC record available at https://lccn.loc.gov/2016053071

ISBN 978-0-451-49696-6
Ebook ISBN 978-0-451-49697-3

Printed in the United States of America

Jacket design by Jenny Carrow
Jacket photographs by (salt shaker) © art-4-art/Getty Images; (pill bottle)
© Billion Photos/Shutterstock
Frontispiece photograph: Deyan Georgiev/Shutterstock

10 9 8 7 6 5 4 3 2 1

First Edition

For my beautiful wife, Megan,

and my wonderful children, Alexander and Emmalyn

CONTENTS

. . . .

Introduction

. . . .

Don't Fear the Shaker

Consider Scandinavian novelist Isak Dinesen's famous line, "The cure for anything is salt water: sweat, tears or the sea."

There's poetic truth in this, but it also speaks to our biological reality as humans. Our physical inner world was born of the sea, and we carry the saltiness of the ocean inside us. Salt is an essential nutrient that our body depends on to live. Its proper balance is an equilibrium that our bodies strive to return us to, again and again.

But over the past century, our culture has defied this biological drive, has smeared the urge for salt as a self-destructive "addiction." We've all heard the guidelines. We know that we're supposed to eat low-saturated-fat diets, say no to cigarettes, go for a jog, learn to relax—and dramatically cut down on salt. This list of admonishments certainly gets a lot of things right. But there's one big problem with it: most of us don't need to eat low-salt diets. In fact, for most of us, *more* salt would be better for our health rather than less.

Meanwhile, the white crystal we've demonized all these years has been taking the fall for another, one so sweet that we refused to believe it wasn't benign. A white crystal that, consumed in excess, can lead to high blood pressure, cardiovascular disease, and chronic kidney disease: not salt, but sugar.

Thankfully, the mainstream press is starting to catch on that sugar is a wolf in sheep's clothing, with low-sugar diets rising in popularity every day. And even fat has been getting a fresh look, as we're now encouraged to seek out the beneficial kinds in fatty fish, avocados, and olives.

So why do we still see labels on salty foods that make the saltshaker look downright toxic? Why do we keep reading fearmongering headlines about salt in mainstream, reputable media, like these?

Eating Too Much Salt Is Killing Us by the Millions
—*Forbes*, March 24, 2013

1.6 Million Heart Disease Deaths Every Year Caused by Eating Too Much Salt
—*Healthline News*, August 14, 2014

U.S. Teens Eat Too Much Salt, Hiking Obesity Risk
—*HealthDay*, February 3, 2014

For the Good of Your Heart, Keep Holding the Salt
—*Harvard Health Blog*, July 11, 2016

The truth is, our most hallowed health institutions cling to outdated, disproven theories about salt—and their resistance to the truth is putting our public health at risk. Until the low-salt dogma is successfully challenged, we'll be stuck in this same perpetual loop that keeps our bodies salt-deprived, sugar-addicted, and ultimately deficient in many critical nutrients. Many of us will continue struggling with insatiable hunger and hold on to weight around the middle despite following recommended lifestyle changes.

If you're diligent about your health, you may have been struggling to achieve the low-salt guidelines that limit you to 2,300 milligrams of sodium (basically 1 teaspoon of salt) per day—or even 1,500 milligrams ($^2/_3$ teaspoon of salt) if you are older, are African American, or have high blood pressure. Indeed, according to the Centers for Disease Control and Prevention (CDC), more than 50 percent of people in the United States are currently monitoring or reducing their sodium intake, and almost 25 percent are being told by a health professional to curb their consumption of sodium.[1]

If you are among them, you may have been buying less-tasty "low sodium" versions of your favorite foods. You may feel a twinge of guilt when you sneak a handful of your partner's popcorn at the movies. You may have picked olives out of your salad and ignored every recipe's call to "salt to taste." Perhaps it's been years since you've had a warm, salty pretzel or a bowl of satisfying puttanesca, full of savory capers, out of fear of those evil grams of sodium.

You may have been mightily struggling to restrict yourself, not knowing that your salt cravings are totally, biologically normal, akin to our thirst for water. Scientists have found that across all populations, when people are left to unrestricted sodium consumption, they tend to settle in at 3,000 to 4,000 milligrams of sodium per day. This amount holds true for people in all hemispheres, all climates, all range of cultures and social backgrounds—when permitted free access to salt, all humans gravitate to the same threshold of salt consumption, a threshold we now know is the sodium-intake range for optimal health.

Your body has been talking to you, and it's time to listen. The good news is, you probably don't need to cut down. In fact, you may need even *more* salt. Instead of ignoring your salt cravings, you should give in to them—they are guiding you to better health.

In these pages, I'm going to set the record straight and upend everyday myths about the supposed negative effects of salt. I'll tell the story of how humans evolved from the briny sea, how our biology shapes our taste for salt—and how this taste is actually an unfailing guide. I'll tell the story of the Salt Wars of the past century—the varying dietary guidelines that have led us so far astray. I'll explain how our essential physiological need for salt is increased by the demands of modern life and how we're actually at a greater risk for salt depletion than ever before. (Two-thirds of the world's population now struggles

with three or more chronic health conditions, many of which increase the risk of low salt levels in the body.) I'll talk about how many
commonly prescribed medications, beloved caffeinated beverages,
and widely touted dietary strategies actually *promote* salt depletion.
I'll examine how many of the negative health effects that have been
blamed on salt are really due to excess *sugar* consumption—and how
eating more salt can be instrumental in breaking the sugar addiction
cycle.

Along the way, I'll also include recommendations for how to use
salt to improve your exercise performance and increase muscle gain,
and how not to fall short in crucial iodine. I'll give specific recommendations on how to strategically increase your intake of the right
kinds of salt, in the amounts *your* body needs (because some people
need more salt than others). You'll learn how eating the salt your
body desires can improve everything from your sleep, energy levels,
and mental focus to your fertility and even sexual performance. Finally, I will cover numerous medications, disease states, and lifestyle
choices that lead to salt wasting, so you can have a better idea if you
are at risk of salt deficit.

As I share these findings, you'll also hear stories from many people, including those struggling with chronic diseases, such as high
blood pressure, heart failure, obesity, or kidney disease, and hard-
charging elite athletes looking for a competitive advantage. You'll
hear about how eating certain kinds of salt—or simply giving in to
salt cravings—helped these people feel healthier, have more energy,
improve athletic performance, resolve long-standing chronic conditions, and even lose weight. People such as AJ, a man in his early
thirties with hypertension who'd been advised to reduce his salt
intake—but found his blood pressure unchanged, his energy levels
plummeting, and vicious headaches recurring. It was only after AJ
reintroduced salt—as much as he wanted—while he reduced his carbohydrate intake that the headaches stopped, he lost 65 pounds, and
he reduced his blood pressure by eighty points. (See AJ's full story on
page 5.) And then, finally, in the last chapter of the book, I'll pull all

of these lessons together and spell out five simple steps to tap into your instinct for salt, get more of the healthiest types of salt, and reverse years of salt imbalances in your body.

In hearing the story about the power of salt, you may find yourself as baffled as I am by the continued resistance to the clear research findings. I'll examine the forces behind this stubborn refusal to accept the truth—and prove that the time for adherence to this long-outdated dogma has come to an end. We need to recognize that science has moved on, and our dietary guidelines need to move on as well. In the names of our hearts, our health, and our happiness, we need to help salt reclaim its rightful and vital place on our table. Simply put, our lives and happiness depend on it.

ADD SALT, REMOVE POUNDS

When my friend Jose Carlos Souto, MD, first treated AJ, he was obese and hypertensive (220/170 mmHg), and had frequent headaches. According to the standard recommendation, AJ had tried to reduce his salt consumption, thinking it would improve his health. Soon thereafter, he began to feel tired all the time and had started to develop unexplained chills every now and then—and his blood pressure remained high. Dr. Souto decided to try another approach—he advised him to go on a low-carb diet and to start eating the amount of salt his body craved. Almost immediately, his energy returned and his chills disappeared. His headaches reduced dramatically. And while his blood pressure remained high for a while, as he began to lose weight, his blood pressure declined at the same time. A year later, he had lost 65 pounds—and, lo and behold, his blood pressure stabilized at 140/90 mmHg, without any medications.

1

. . . .

But Doesn't Salt Cause High Blood Pressure?

For more than forty years, our doctors, the government, and the nation's leading health associations have told us that consuming salt increases blood pressure and thus causes chronic high blood pressure.

Here's the truth: there was never any sound scientific evidence to support this idea. Even back in 1977, when the government's Dietary Goals for the United States recommended that Americans restrict their salt intake, a report from the U.S. Surgeon General admitted there was no evidence that a low-salt diet would prevent the increases in blood pressure that often occur with advancing age.[1] The first systematic review and meta-analysis of the effects of sodium restriction on blood pressure did not occur until 1991, and it was almost entirely based on weak, nonrandomized scientific data—but by then, we had already been telling Americans to cut their salt intake for nearly fifteen years. By that point, those white crystals had already been ingrained into the public's mind as a primary cause of high blood pressure—a message that remains today.

The advice stemmed largely from the most basic of scientific explanations: the "salt–blood pressure hypothesis." This hypothesis held that eating higher levels of salt leads to higher levels of blood pressure—end of story. But that wasn't the full story, of course. As with so many old medical theories, the real story was a bit more complex.

The hypothesis went like this: In the body, we measure blood pressure in two different ways. The top number of a typical blood pressure reading is your *systolic* blood pressure, the pressure in your arteries during contraction of your heart. The bottom number is your *diastolic* blood pressure, the pressure in your arteries when your heart is relaxed. When we eat salt, so the theory goes, we also get thirsty—so we drink more water. In the salt–high blood pressure hypothesis, that excess salt then causes the body to hold on to that increased water, in order to dilute the saltiness of the blood. Then, the resulting increased blood volume would automatically lead to higher blood pressure.

That's the theory, anyway. Makes sense, right?

All of this *did* make sense, in theory, and for a while there was some circumstantial evidence supporting this claim. Data was gathered on salt intake and blood pressures in various populations, and correlations were seen in some cases. But even if those correlations were consistent, as we all know, correlation does not equal causation—just because one thing (salt) may sometimes lead to another thing (higher blood pressure), which happens to correlate with another thing (cardiovascular events), that does not necessarily prove that the first thing *caused* the third thing.

Sure enough, data that conflicted with the salt–blood pressure theory continued to be published right along with data that supported it. A heated debate raged in the scientific community about whether salt induced chronically elevated blood pressure (hypertension) versus a fleeting, inconsequential rise in blood pressure, with advocates and skeptics on both sides. In fact, compared to any other nutrient, even cholesterol or saturated fat, salt has caused the most controversy. And once we got on that salt–high blood pressure train, it was hard to get off. Governments and health agencies had taken a stance on salt, and to admit that they were wrong would cause them to lose face. They continued the same low-salt mantra, refusing to overturn their premature verdict on salt until they were presented with overwhelming evidence to the contrary. No one was willing to get off the train until there was definitive evidence that their presumptions were wrong—instead of asking, "Did we ever have any evidence to recommend sodium restriction in the first place?"

We believed so strongly in sodium restriction because we believed so strongly in blood pressure as a metric of health. Low-salt advocates posit that even a one-point reduction in blood pressure (if translated to millions of people) would actually equal a reduction in strokes and heart attacks. But evidence in the medical literature suggests that approximately 80 percent of people with normal blood pressure (less than 120/80 mmHg) are not sensitive to the blood-pressure-raising effects of salt *at all*. Among those with prehypertension (a precursor to high blood pressure), roughly 75 percent are not sensitive to salt. And even among those with full-blown hypertension, about 55 percent are totally immune to salt's effects on blood pressure.[2]

That's right: even among those with the *highest* blood pressure, about half are not at all affected by salt.

The stringent low-salt guidelines were based on a guess: we essentially gambled that the small benefits to blood pressure that we see in some patients would extend to large benefits for the whole population. And while taking that gamble, we glossed over the most important point: *why* salt may increase blood pressure in *some* people but not in others. Had we focused on that, we would've realized that fixing the underlying issue—which has nothing to do with eating too much salt—completely fixes one's "salt sensitivity." We also presumed that blood pressure, a fleeting measurement known to fluctuate depending on many health factors, was *always* impacted by salt. And because of that baseless certainty, we presumed that overconsumption of salt would *logically* result in dire health outcomes, such as strokes and heart attacks.

Our mistake came from taking such a small sample of people— unethically small!—and wildly extrapolating their benefits from low-salt eating without ever mentioning the risks. Instead, we focused on those extremely minuscule reductions in blood pressure, completely disregarding the numerous other health risks caused by low salt intake—including several side effects that actually *magnify* our risk of heart disease—such as increased heart rate; compromised kidney function and adrenal insufficiency; hypothyroidism; higher triglyceride, cholesterol, and insulin levels; and, ultimately, insulin resistance, obesity, and type 2 diabetes.

Perhaps most illustrative of this willful disregard for risk is the case of heart rate. Heart rate is proven to increase on a low-salt diet. This harmful effect occurs in nearly everyone who restricts his or her salt intake. Although this effect is documented more thoroughly in the medical literature, no food ad or dietary guideline says, "A low-salt diet can increase your risk of elevated heart rate." And what has a bigger impact on your health: a one-point reduction in blood pressure or a four-beat-per-minute increase in heart rate? (In chapter 4, I'll take a closer look at what these metrics mean and I'll let you decide.)

If our bodies allowed us to isolate each of these risks, we might be able to say for certain that one or another is most important. But when you combine all of the *known* dangers of salt restriction, it's easy to see that the harms far outweigh any possible benefits. In other words, we've focused on just one metric that *might* change with a low-salt diet—blood pressure—but completely disregarded all the other harmful effects in the process.

Now that we can recognize our folly, we've come to a moment in our nation's public health when we need to ask ourselves: Have we subjected generations of people—especially those whose health was already compromised—to a "treatment" that may have escalated their health decline?

This question becomes increasingly urgent as the stresses of the modern world inflict a compounded toll on our bodies. In addition to the salt we lose by following our low-carb, ketogenic, or paleo diets, we're also taking more medications that cause salt loss; we're enduring more damage to the intestine that causes decreased salt absorption (including Crohn's disease, ulcerative colitis, irritable bowel syndrome [IBS], and leaky gut); and we're doing more damage to the kidneys by eating more refined carbohydrates and sugar (decreasing the kidneys' ability to retain salt).

Recent research even suggests that chronic salt depletion may be a factor in what endocrinologists term "internal starvation." When you start restricting your salt intake, the body starts to panic. One of the body's defense mechanisms is to increase insulin levels, because insulin helps the kidneys retain more sodium. Unfortunately, high insulin levels also "lock" energy into your fat cells, so that you have trouble breaking down stored fat into fatty acids or stored protein into amino acids for energy. When your insulin levels are elevated, the only macronutrient that you can efficiently utilize for energy is carbohydrate.[3]

See where this is headed?

You start craving sugar and refined carbs like crazy, because your body believes carbohydrate is your only viable energy source. And, as the now-familiar story goes, the more refined carbs you eat, the more refined carbs you tend to crave. This overeating of processed carbs and high-sugar foods virtually ensures fat cell accumulation, weight gain, insulin resistance, and eventually type 2 diabetes.

What's clear is that we have been focusing on the wrong white crystal all along. We demonized sodium before we had the evidence. And our health has been paying the price ever since. Had we left salt on the table, our health problems in general—and especially those pertaining to sugar—might be a little less dramatic.

It's time to set the record straight. It's time to drop the guilt, grab the shaker, and enjoy salt again!

Time for the Truth

I've always been very athletic, running cross-country and wrestling in high school, so I know a great deal about how nutrition (or lack thereof) impacts performance. All those afternoons of running, and then spending my days as a wrestler in the sauna to lose weight, made me appreciate how important salt is for athletes.

After high school, I graduated from the University at Buffalo with my Doctor of Pharmacy degree and began to work in the community as a pharmacist. I became even more interested in salt when I found out that one of my patients was complaining of fatigue, dizziness, and lethargy. While puzzling this out with her, I remembered that she was on a medication (an antidepressant called sertraline) that can increase the risk of low sodium levels in the blood. When I put together her doctor's instructions to cut her salt intake with the additional prescription of a diuretic, I immediately suspected that she was dehydrated because of salt depletion and that her blood sodium levels were low. I suggested that she might need to start eating more salt but advised her to get her blood sodium levels tested first to confirm my suspicions.

Sure enough, her sodium levels were extremely low. Her doctor cut the dose of her diuretic in half and told her to eat more salt. After that, it wasn't long before all of her symptoms went away. The following week, she came into the pharmacy to tell me that I was right and that I helped to dramatically improve the quality of her life—just about the best thing any person in a medical field can hear. I was extremely relieved and encouraged that the solution to her symptoms was so simple, so inexpensive, and so immediately effective.

That experience prompted me to take a deeper look into the low-salt guidelines. The deeper I looked, the more I could see that maybe the advice we had been giving people, to cut their salt intake, wasn't correct after all. Around the same time, in 2013, I took a position as a cardiovascular research scientist at Saint Luke's Mid America Heart Institute. After joining Saint Luke's, I published nearly two hundred medical papers in the scientific literature, many relating to the impact of salt and sugar on health. Based on these academic publications, that same year I was offered a position as the associate editor of BMJ Open Heart, an official journal of the British Cardiovascular Society.

In total, I've spent nearly a decade examining the research on salt and working with clinicians to untangle the complexity of our salt intake and get to the heart of the issue. Should we do away with these outdated restrictions? Who really needs less salt—and who needs more? How much—and what kinds—are optimal? And perhaps most exciting, how might increasing our salt intake actually help us turn back the tide of obesity and stem the rising epidemic of type 2 diabetes that threatens to overwhelm our nation, and the entire world?

We can start by telling the truth:

Low salt is miserable.

Low salt is dangerous.

Our bodies evolved to need salt.

Low-salt guidelines are based on inherited "wisdom," not scientific fact.

All the while, the real culprit has been sugar.

And finally: salt may be one solution to—rather than a cause of—our nation's chronic disease crises.

Your body drives you to eat several grams of salt (around 8–10 grams, equal to 3,000–4,000 milligrams of sodium) every day to remain in homeostasis, an optimal state in which you put the least amount of stress on the body. But you could literally live the rest of your life—and probably a much longer one—if you never ingested another gram of added sugar.

Now, I understand that it will take a bit of time to unlearn years of indoctrination about the evils of salt—which is why I wrote this book. In these chapters, you'll learn the entire story. (By the end, in chapters 7 and 8, you will find specific recommendations for how you can find and implement your ideal salt intake.) But that understanding begins with reeducation about the myriad ways our lives can be healthier, stronger, and longer when we welcome salt back into our lives.

If salt has always played such a fundamental role in human health, how did we ever begin to doubt it? Perhaps salt's ubiquity was one of the factors in its downfall; perhaps we simply took it for granted. In order to understand how we could have gone so far off course, we first have to understand the critical role salt has always played in human health, from the moment life slithered out of the sea right up until the birth of modern medicine. By looking closely at salt's crucial role in our past, we can start to restore its tarnished reputation and honor salt's place in our future.

We Are Salty Folk

We are essentially salty people.

We cry salt, we sweat salt, and the cells in our bodies are bathed in salty fluids. Without salt we would not be able to live.

Just a small dash of salt can take a bland dish and heighten all of its flavors, making it taste extraordinary. Salt knocks out bitterness and makes food taste sweeter, reducing the need for sugar. And just as much as we relish the satisfaction and savory heartiness that salt adds to our food, salt plays a fundamental role in dozens of critical functions in our bodies.

Salt is needed to maintain the optimal amount of blood in our bodies; it's even needed by the heart to pump blood throughout our bodies. Salt is essential for digestion, cell-to-cell communication, bone formation and strength, and prevention of dehydration. Sodium is also critical to reproduction, the proper functioning of cells and muscles, and the optimal transmission of nerve impulses to and from organs such as the heart and brain. Indeed, our bodies rely on elements called electrolytes—such as sodium, potassium, magnesium, and calcium—in our bodily fluids to help carry out electrical impulses that control many of our bodies' functions. Without an adequate sodium intake, our blood volume goes down, which could lead to the shutting down of certain organs, such as the brain and kidneys.

Simply put, if we eliminated all sodium from our diets, we would die.

Our brain and body automatically determine how much sodium we eat, reabsorb, and excrete. The ability of our body to conserve salt and water is thought to be controlled by our hypothalamus, a part of our so-called reptilian brain that both receives and transmits signals that drive us to crave salt or feel thirsty.

Those signals, if we honor them, lead us to naturally create optimal levels of water and salt in the body—because those powerful instinctual drives are a direct result of evolutionary facts of life. The first living creatures on the planet were bathed in seawater, and when they came onto land, they took salt from the ocean with them.[1] And, today, millions of years later, the makeup of our human body fluids still mimics that of the ancient ocean.

Out of the Ocean

The ocean covers 71 percent of the earth's surface, but because of its massive volume, the ocean also makes up 99 percent of the earth's total living space.[2] Sodium chloride, aka salt, constitutes 90 percent of the entire ocean's mineral content,[3] the same percentage of mineral content found in our blood. The only difference between the two is in concentration—the ocean is four to five times as salty as our own blood (around 3.5 percent NaCl versus 0.82 percent NaCl).[4] Besides the ocean, salt can also be found in smaller seas, rock salt, brackish water, salt licks, and even rainwater. The vast amount of salt we find in numerous areas around the world only underscores the importance of salt to all forms of life.

The similarity between the mineral content and concentration of our own blood and seawater has been known for decades.[5] Cells can't survive outside a narrow range of electrolyte levels in the extracellular fluid that bathes them. In order for a species to leave the ocean and survive on land, several salt-regulating systems had to develop and evolve. Those systems operate all over our bodies, including in our skin, adrenal glands, and kidneys.

The precise ionic calibrations that facilitate cell life have not changed substantially since the beginning of life itself.[6] Even now, our bodies retain salt in times of scarcity and excrete excess salt when we don't need it. This ability to regulate the amount of salt in our bodies and to seek it out in times of need has allowed us to survive and thrive in almost every type of geographical region in the world— but, in essence, our blood still reflects the ancient ocean where life began and from which it evolved.

Compared to the dramatic changes in the form, structure, and function of organs that occurred during vertebrate evolution, the fact that the electrolyte makeup of the extracellular fluid has generally remained constant[7] suggests that salt balance is an evolutionary adaptation. This adaptation remains tightly regulated for sustaining life for all vertebrates, including marine and freshwater fish and turtles, reptiles, birds, amphibians, and, yes, mammals.[8] That fact is foundational to the theory that all animals—including humans—are thought to have evolved from creatures that originated in the ocean.[9]

Once sea invertebrates developed a closed circulatory system, they would have needed to evolve organs called kidneys to help them reabsorb and excrete salt and water (among other things). Until then, the salty ocean would have been integrated into the invertebrate itself. From an evolutionary perspective, then, the kidneys likely first evolved *in* the sea and would therefore consider salt a friend, not an enemy. This fact seems to be lost in our current debate about optimal salt intake.

An organism's ability to retain and excrete salt is critical in order to provide the proper cell function and hydration that sustains life. There is no better example of this than fish that are able to live in both freshwater and salt water. Most of these fish can actively reabsorb or excrete sodium via their gills, allowing for drastic environmental change in saltiness.[10] The gills of these fish serve much like the kidneys of a human, reabsorbing or excreting sodium depending on whether they have too much or too little salt in their body, thereby helping to maintain normal electrolyte and water balance. Another evolutionary adaptation to maintain salt and water homeostasis is the heavy armor-plating seen in freshwater reptiles. This adaptation allows maintenance of normal electrolyte and fluid balance, as the shell counters the drastic difference in osmotic stress of living in a freshwater environment—where the concentration of salt is much less than that of blood.[11]

Despite significant changes in the saltiness of the animals' environments, their organs continued to evolve in order to maintain normal salt concentrations, and hence water balance, in the blood, no matter where their travels took them—even as they took those first critical slithers onto land.

Crawling Up on Shore

Tetrapods, the first four-limbed vertebrates, are thought to be the last common ancestor of amphibians, reptiles, and mammals. These animals were first able to leave the seas by swallowing air into their gut.[12] Once these creatures were on land, their kidneys had to adapt from living in the salty environment of the sea to one that was relatively salt-scarce.

While there are many theories about the origin of land-based animals and the rise of vertebrates from invertebrates, our kidneys and our salt cravings are big clues that we more likely evolved from marine animals rather than freshwater animals.[13] If we did come from the sea, the evolutionary ability to retain sodium would have been a requirement, one that allowed the maintenance of blood pressure and circulation of blood through the tissues once on land.[14] These animals, once bathed in salt water, were now faced with the relative salt scarcity of the desert, rain forest, mountains, and other nonmarine environments. Thus, not only was it important to retain salt, but a "hunger" for salt would have evolved in these animals to ensure that their needs were met. This "hunger" would provide a physiological signal—an appetite—to seek out salt whenever a deficit was on the horizon. Their brand-new closed circulatory systems would give them an enhanced ability to maintain sodium and water homeostasis, mostly due to the evolution of the kidneys, bladder, skin, intestines, and other endocrine glands not present in ancient marine inverte-brates.[15]

In the animal kingdom, there are no dietary guidelines, of course—no medical directives to create a conscious effort to restrict salt intake. Indeed, many animals (especially those hunting in the sea) ingest large amounts of salt simply as a matter of course during their daily lives. Take, for example, reptiles, birds, and marine mammals, such as the sea lion, sea otter, seal, walrus, and polar bear, that hunt prey living in the ocean. These animals take in large amounts of salt, both from the animal itself and from salt water, during a kill, particularly if they eat oceanic invertebrates, which have the same salt concentration as the ocean.[16] For these marine mammals, the salt content of their blood is not very different from that of terrestrial mammals[17]—and since they are ingesting sea water, which is four to five times as salty as their blood, that salt must be excreted via their kidneys.

Or, to say it bluntly: their kidneys must be able to excrete *massive* amounts of salt.

This basic physiology of the kidneys is the same in humans. In fact, research has shown that patients with normal blood pressure and kidney function can easily excrete *ten times* as much salt as we normally consume in a day.[18] The reason why humans cannot solely live on seawater is not that our kidneys cannot handle excreting the high salt content—it's that in order to do so, water must leave with it, which would eventually cause dehydration (and eventual death!). But if we had enough access to freshwater to replace what is lost during the excretion of that salt, humans would absolutely be able to drink seawater.

Almost without exception, salt and water regulation is a well-adapted survival mechanism for nearly all animals—and this includes all primates, including humans.

Prehuman Primates

Even today, most people believe that prehuman primates (such as orangutans, monkeys, baboons, and macaques) subsisted mainly on fruit and terrestrial vegetation. Thus, one group of scientists has insisted that our prehuman bodies evolved on a low-salt diet. But that is clearly not the case.

Millions of years ago, climate changes that featured intense dry seasons were thought to have forced nonhuman primates to seek out wetlands.[19] Their diet would have consisted of aquatic vegetation, with a sodium content five hundred times that of terrestrial plants.[20] This may also be when nonhuman primates started eating meat, which they would have first encountered when fish and aquatic invertebrates were trapped in aquatic vegetation—providing primates with the original seafood salad.[21] Once these foods were "inadvertently" eaten, nonhuman primates probably got a taste for them and started seeking them out deliberately. Their first fish were thought to have been easier prey, such as catfish that were injured, washed ashore, or trapped in shallow ponds. (Catfish were plentiful where ancestral primates and early humans roamed, making this a plausible notion.)

This dietary switch—toward consuming more fat and omega-3s— certainly makes sense for its potential to foster the development of a larger (more human-sized) brain. Dozens of nonhuman primates have been reported to eat fish and other aquatic fauna that would have supplied their diet with ample amounts of salt.[22] They would have encountered such things as shark eggs, shrimp, crabs, mussels, razor clams, snails, octopus, oysters and other shelled invertebrates, tree frogs, invertebrates in the river mud, snapping turtle eggs, water beetles, limpets, tadpoles, sand-hoppers, seal-lice, and earthworms.[23] These abounded at seashores and in swamps, freshwater and marine water, and other tropical and temperate locations. Based on this list, it's obvious that the diet of prehuman primates (and thus early humans) would not have been low in salt; in fact, it could have been extremely *high* in salt.

The taste for fish and other aquatic creatures may have led these prehuman primates to begin deliberately trying to catch fish by hand and eventually using tools such as sticks, sand, and food to catch fish—which represented a huge leap forward in cognitive development. Think of that twist of fate: eating fish by happenstance may have enabled early primate brains to develop the intellect to actively catch fish through the use of tools. Exactly how they were able to obtain these salty creatures is more of a mystery, but it is thought that they used rocks to crack shells open and tapped on bamboo to find frogs living inside it. At least five other species, beyond orangutans, have been found to use tools to obtain fish and other salty aquatic prey. Thereafter, hominins—both modern and extinct humans— would have used primate fish-catching practices.[24]

Early Humans

Intriguingly, the emergence of tool-assisted fish catching in early *Homo* dates to around 2.4 million years ago. Primate fish-eating habits suggest that hominins would have also started eating aquatic plants first, then accidentally sampled the aquatic animals clinging to their nightly feeding, and, having acquired a taste for a newfound meat, eventually transitioned to catching fish and other aquatic prey.[25] Some researchers assert that an early human, *Paranthropus boisei*, and early *Homo* dug into wetlands to add vertebrates and invertebrates to what had previously been their predominantly plant-based diet. These aquatic animal foods yield plenty of salt and novel, high-quality nutrients, such as docosahexaenoic acid (DHA). Similar to how these essential fatty acids may have led to brain growth in prehuman primates, DHA allowed for the brain to increase in size in early humans.[26]

The fact that DHA is important for the growth of the human

SALT HELPS HER BREATHE

One of my friends and colleagues, Sean Lucan, MD, MPH, an associate professor in the Department of Family and Social Medicine at the Montefiore Medical Center of Albert Einstein College of Medicine, told me that he has completely changed his take on salt. "I used to be very anti-salt. I didn't own a saltshaker and I advised my patients not to use salt in their cooking or on their food," he recalls. "I bought into the transitive argument that salt equaled high blood pressure in the short term, and heart attacks and strokes down the road. But as I became increasingly interested in nutrition and I started to look at the evidence, I became increasingly skeptical of the benefits of my own salt avoidance and of the advice I was giving my patients."

A few years ago, Sean went to a symposium on nutrition and cooking at the Culinary Institute of America, which he credits with changing his perspective: "I came to appreciate salt as a culinary ingredient, and I began using salt in my own cooking. The results were immediate, dramatic, and fantastic. I was cooking only real food. And now that real food tasted really good."

His family was thrilled by the way salt made all their food taste better, and none suffered any untoward health consequences as a result of greater sodium intake. He recalled this experience when he became involved in the care of a woman with late-stage congestive heart failure who was on the strictest regimen of sodium restriction. "All she wanted was to taste her food. But her doctors had banned salt from her table and her family had removed it from the house," he recalls. "As she was approaching the ultimate end, I finally convinced her family to allow her some salt. They were reluctant, fearing she would decompensate." But recognizing her desperation and not wanting to deny her such an earnest wish, they agreed.

"And you know what? She did better. No, her heart failure didn't resolve—but her blood pressure didn't suffer, she stopped gasping for air, and she didn't have to return to the hospital as had become a routine. Moreover, she enjoyed her remaining meals and the remaining days of her life, as opposed to suffering unnecessarily in hard-to-rationalize deprivation.

"I still have a picture of one of her great-grandsons sitting on her lap. He is a few years older now, and unlike most other children his age, he only eats real food. And he salts his food according to his own taste. And he is healthy and well, and an example to us all."

brain creates the unavoidable suggestion that aquatic foods—and the hunger for salt that drew our ancestors to them—were an important player in how the human brain evolved into what it is today.[27] Terrestrial plants are low in DHA, which suggests that this transition to aquatic vegetation and prey was essential to increasing our brain size.[28] Imagine: our hunger for salt may have played a role in early humans' great leap forward.

Even early humans who lived far from the ocean's brackish waters had this hunger for salt. Data suggests that early humans roaming East Africa's noncoastal regions between 1.4 and 2.4 million years ago may have consumed a diet extremely high in salt. An ancient ancestor to humans known as "Nutcracker Man" was said to have lived on large amounts of tiger nuts.[29] The fossils of this early human, discovered in 1959 in Tanzania, feature strong jaw muscles as well as wear and tear on molars, indicative of a diet high in tiger nuts. Tiger nuts are *extremely* high in salt (up to 3,383 milligrams of sodium per 100 grams, the average amount of sodium we modern humans eat in an entire day).[30] Just a handful (3 ounces) of these nutlike tubers would have provided an entire day's worth of sodium in today's world.

Nutcracker Man did not live by nuts alone. He also survived on a diet largely composed of grasshoppers. A close relative of the grass-hopper, the cricket contains a very good amount of sodium (about 152 milligrams of sodium per five crickets).[31] Most likely, certain insects are so high in sodium because it allows them to move and fly faster and thus avoid being eaten by their brethren.[32] Scientists have observed that sodium deficiency can lead to cannibalism in insects (and probably other animals, too).[33] The theory goes that the animals instinctively know that salt is contained within blood, interstitial fluid, skin, muscle, and other parts of their bodies. Not surprisingly, experts believe humans have been getting protein and micronutrients from wild insects for several millennia—and continue to do so to this day, particularly in parts of Africa, Asia, and Mexico.[34]

The Case Is Clear

From an evolutionary standpoint, evidence does not suggest that we evolved on a low-salt diet. Instead, much of our evolutionary theory seems to support the fact that we evolved on a high-salt diet. So where does this persistent misconception about our original diet come from?

The idea that our human ancestors consumed very little salt, generally less than 1,500 milligrams of sodium per day, is both old and current.[35] Some of the debate about evolutionary diet seems to stem from one influential paper on the topic, which was published in 1985 in the *New England Journal of Medicine*, one of the world's most prestigious medical journals. The authors of this paper estimated that during the Paleolithic era (from about 2.6 million years ago until about 10,000 years ago), our intake of sodium was just 700 milligrams per day.[36] But this figure was based on the sodium content of select land animals (and only the sodium content of the meat) as well as land plants available to hunter-gatherers. This estimate does not include the sodium that would have been obtained from tiger nuts, insects, or aquatic vegetation or prey, nor does it include the other large stores of sodium found in animals besides the meat, such as that found in the skin, interstitial fluid, blood, and bone marrow (which we know hunter-gatherers *did* eat). We can't forget that, aside from their meat, animals themselves (muscle, organs, viscera, skin, blood) are extremely good sources of salt. For example, muscle contains approximately 1,150 milligrams of sodium per kilogram. Australian Aborigines would eat 2 to 3 kilograms of meat per sitting during a kill.[37] This is equal to 3,450 milligrams of sodium per day, the exact amount of sodium that current-day Americans consume (when they're not straining to achieve the low-salt guidelines, that is!). Organs of animals are even higher in salt than meat: just 10 ounces of bison ribs (about one-quarter of a kilogram) provides 1,500 milligrams of sodium, the same amount in just 13.5 ounces of bison kidney or 2 pounds of bison liver. And remember, this doesn't even include the salt that is found in the skin, interstitial fluid, blood, and bone marrow.

Early humans probably got salt in other ways as well. Some would have also eaten soil, as is still done by Kikuyu women of Africa, who are known to make dishes from sodium-rich soil.[38] Our ancestors also likely had salt licks and drank rainwater, providing clear evidence that previous estimates of sodium intake during our evolution are most likely drastic underestimations.

But alas, the mantra has always been that the strict vegetarian diet of our early ancestors only provides around 230 milligrams of sodium per day, and that even a carnivorous diet only provides around 1,400 milligrams of sodium. These low estimates led most experts to believe that our current salt intake is two to twenty times what our ancestors would have consumed. And if we didn't eat that much salt during our evolution, then our current intake can't be good for us! (Or so the mantra goes.)

No one truly knows how much salt our Paleolithic ancestors ate or how much salt our human brain evolved on—but it's probably much more than what most experts think. Some experts believe that 45 to

60 percent of our Paleolithic ancestors' calories came from animal foods[39] that are naturally high in salt.

Humans Have Always Needed Salt

We know salt was important to early humans, reflecting and mimicking the marine environment from which we came. But we've supposedly evolved far beyond that stage—so what does salt do for us now?

Salt (aka sodium chloride, or NaCl) is the white substance that we all know from the dinner table. NaCl turns into electrolytes once it is dissolved in the blood and other bodily fluids, forming the positively charged sodium ion (Na+) and the negatively charged chloride ion (Cl–). Na+ is the main positively charged electrolyte known as a cation (pronounced cat-eye-on) that makes up the fluid that bathes our cells; chloride is the main negatively charged electrolyte known as an anion (pronounced an-eye-on) in our blood. Na+ and Cl– are the electrolytes of highest concentration in our blood as compared to any other electrolyte (such as potassium, magnesium, or calcium).

Iodine is also a mineral, like sodium and chloride, but it is only found in trace amounts in the body. Despite being a trace mineral, iodine is essential to our entire body's health. Iodine is the main building block of our thyroid hormones, with three iodine atoms making up the thyroid hormone T3 (triiodothyronine) and four iodine atoms making up T4 (thyroxine). A deficiency in iodine decreases the body's production of T3 and T4 and can enlarge the thyroid tissue, causing goiter and possibly leading to underactive (hypothyroid) or overactive (hyperthyroid) thyroid function.

The water and sodium levels in our body are constantly balancing each other out, a process known as osmoregulation. Whenever there is an increase in sodium concentration in the blood, the kidneys simply reabsorb less sodium, the excess gets excreted in our urine, and the body maintains a normal serum sodium level in the blood. This mechanism helps to prevent cellular damage from fluid shifting in and out of cells.

If blood sodium levels drop too low, water from the blood will go into our tissue cells in order to increase the level of sodium in the blood back to normal, but this fluid shift can lead to cellular swelling. If the sodium level in the blood goes up, water will be pulled out of the tissue cells and into the blood, in order to lower sodium levels back to normal—but this can cause cellular shrinkage. Both cellular expansion and cellular shrinkage can be extremely harmful, which is why our body will do anything to keep a normal sodium level in the blood and why salt intake and balance are so tightly regulated. If our body were not able to do this, a low blood sodium level could lead to too much water in the brain, eventually causing death.

One evolutionary adaptation that allowed us to better balance salt once we were on land was the transformation in the production of adrenal hormones. Lower vertebrates inhabiting salty environments produce cortisol and corticosterone, whereas nonaquatic land-dwelling animals evolved to produce corticosterone and aldosterone.[40] Humans then evolved to produce cortisol and aldosterone. These adrenal hormones are critical in our fight-or-flight nervous system response (cortisol) as well as our salt balance (cortisol and aldosterone).

Cortisol, perhaps the most famous "stress hormone," is the primary glucocorticoid produced by our adrenal glands during times of stress. Cortisol also seems to be involved in the release of sodium from our skin stores to aid us during stressful times. Remember how insects can apparently fly faster if they are saltier? Well, the same thing may occur with humans who are trying to avoid being eaten by a lion. Aldosterone, another hormone released by our adrenal glands, socks sodium away into our skin and allows us to reabsorb more salt from the kidneys in times of deficit or need. So aldosterone is a "salt storer" whereas cortisol seems to be a "salt releaser," with the interplay of both hormones helping to determine our overall salt status.

Another physiological regulator of our salt status is something known as a volume sensor, or receptor, which is found in our carotid arteries and the aorta. These receptors sense pressure changes that trigger signals in the brain, causing the kidneys to either retain or excrete more salt and water, depending on body sodium stores.[41] On average, our kidneys may filter between 3.2 and 3.6 *pounds* of salt (1.28 and 1.44 pounds of sodium) per day.[42] This is about 150 times the amount of salt we ingest per day. To put this into perspective, most health agencies tell us that consuming just 6 grams of salt (around 2,300 milligrams of sodium or 1 teaspoon of salt) is too high, yet our kidneys filter this amount of salt *every five minutes.*

The salt restriction recommendations hardly make sense from a physiological viewpoint, but seeing these numbers helps to put things further into perspective. The amount of salt we eat per day is truly a drop in the bucket compared to the amount that the kidneys filter on a daily basis. In fact, the stress on our kidneys mainly comes from having to conserve salt and *reabsorb* all of the 3.2 to 3.6 pounds of salt that we filter every day.[43] This reabsorption requires us to use up adenosine triphosphate (ATP), the energy created from the food we ingest that's utilized by our cells to facilitate many bodily functions. Our sodium pump uses approximately 70 percent of the basal energy expended by the kidneys,[44] making a low-salt diet an energy hog and a tremendous stress to the kidneys. This is one way that low-salt diets can lead to weight gain, by slowly depleting our energy stores and leading us to become more sedentary. What organism would want to move (and sweat out precious sodium) when it has too little salt to begin with?

Similar to the way a low-salt diet depletes the energy of the kidneys, it does the same to the heart.[45] When we restrict our salt intake, our heart rate goes up, reducing our blood and oxygen circulation throughout our body and increasing the heart's need for oxygen.[46] Any one of these effects, all produced by a low-salt diet, could increase our risk of having a heart attack.

Getting enough salt is critical for so many things. Diarrhea, vomiting, and sweating can lead to salt deficit. A salt deficit can reduce speed and endurance as well as thermoregulation in athletes.[47] Getting enough salt creates the right fluid-sodium balance, so it prevents dehydration, low blood pressure, dizziness, falls, and cognitive impairment. And perhaps most importantly for the fate of the human race, salt is essential for reproduction.

Salt and Sex

One of salt's most intriguing properties is its importance for many facets of reproduction—from sexual desire and procreation to gestation and lactation[48]—and this connection has been known at least since the time of the ancient Greeks. In the Aegean world, Aphrodite, the goddess of love, encourages mating and reproduction and prevents infertility. Aphrodite is commonly depicted as having been born from the salty sea foam and known as the "salt born." She is thought to symbolize the "generative" power of salt and the ancient Greeks' belief in the origin of mankind from salted foam.[49]

Greek thinker and philosopher Aristotle observed this power among the agricultural animals of the time, stating that "sheep are in a better condition by keeping their hydro-mineral balance under control. The animals that drink saline water can copulate earlier. Salt must be given to them before they give birth and during lactation." Aristotle's contemporaries knew that animals that ate a lot of salt produced more milk—and salt made animals lusty and eager to mate.[50]

Today, farmers see these same effects among modern livestock animals. Cutting sodium has been found to reduce birth weights and litter size.[51] Reducing the level of salt in feed for lactating sows doubles their average time from weaning their offspring to fertility; it also reduces successful mating in female adult pigs. And in mice, sodium deficiency has also been found to trigger reproduction failure.

In all settings, when animals become sodium deficient, they go out of their way to find this vital mineral. A yen for salt drives the elephants of Kenya to walk into the pitch-black caves of Mount Elgon to lick sodium sulfate off the cave walls. Elephants in the Gabon who are deprived of salt uproot entire trees to get at the sodium-rich soil under the roots. Even gorillas have been known to follow elephants to eat the salt-rich soil and chew on rotting wood, to eat the salty microbes.[52] Monkeys that groom one another don't do so to eat fleas, as is commonly presumed—they do it to eat each other's salty skin secretions.[53] Many animals participate in puddling to get salt from soil[54] and will even drink urine to obtain salt. *Papilio polytes*, a type of swallowtail butterfly, has been found to drink seawater at low tide to help meet salt requirements.[55]

A low-salt diet seems to act like a natural contraceptive in both animals and humans, and in both males and females. A low-salt diet causes a reduced sex drive; reduced likelihood of getting pregnant; reduced litter size (in animals) and weight of infants; and increased erectile dysfunction, fatigue, sleep problems, and age at which women become fertile.[56] The low-salt-eating Yanomamo Indians average only one live birth every four to six years, despite being sexually active and not using contraception.[57] Research has found that women with salt-wasting kidneys due to a congenital adrenal problem have a decreased fertility and childbirth rate.[58]

Modern medicine diverted us from our evolutionary path when it decided that salt was a toxic, addictive, nonessential food additive. The seeds of this destructive myth were sown one hundred years ago, but we are still bearing the costs now.

The War against Salt—and How We Demonized the Wrong White Crystal

When it comes to our current salt intake, we may be guilty as charged—we *do* tend to eat more salt than the *minimum* amount we need to live.

On the surface, this excess can seem like a convincing argument for cutting down on salt. Why eat more than necessary? But just like any nutrient, salt has an optimal level of intake that provides longevity and ideal health—but that optimal level comes with both an upper *and* a lower limit.

Think about it: no one would think to recommend an intake of calcium or vitamin D that is a *minimal* amount to live. The consequences of getting too little are well known, such as a higher risk of osteoporosis and rickets. The concern is rarely about getting too much of either—but rather, too little. Much less is known about the harms of not eating enough salt—and in that vacuum, the fear that eating too much would lead to "sodium-induced" hypertension prevailed. We now know just how foolish, shortsighted, and dangerous that lack of awareness has been.

For years, in order to gain support for salt restriction, many low-salt advocates forcefully and relentlessly argued that the increased intake of salt was paralleled by a rise in hypertension and cardiovascular disease around the world.[1] We have been told that for millions of years humans would have consumed at most only around 1 gram of salt (around 400 milligrams of sodium) per day, a view that is still shared by many today—despite the clear evolutionary evidence you read about in the last chapter.[2] In fact, if we suspend our assumptions and just look at the historical data, we see that the exact opposite was true: as hypertension and chronic disease were on the rise in the Western world, salt intake was already on the decline.

How did these glaring contradictions—that humans throughout history consumed only a fraction of today's salt intake, that salt causes high blood pressure, and that high blood pressure causes heart disease—take hold of the medical field so completely? And how have they maintained their iron grip for almost a century?

The truth is, a small number of emphatically held assumptions derailed scientific progress for decades—if not generations. To trace the roots of these beliefs and find the truths behind them, let's first look at how humans interacted with salt as civilization unfolded. By understanding the history and psychology of our relationship with salt, we can trace the progression from a few researchers' mistaken assumptions and how—through a lethal combination of inertia, publication bias, and nefarious interests motivated by the food industry—those assumptions became established medical dogma and public health guidelines.

Mining for White Gold

Humans have been consciously producing salt, by scraping salt from dried desert lake beds or mining salt from the earth, for at least eight thousand years.[3] Salt mining started in China but spread to various regions around the world—including Egypt, Jerusalem, Italy, Spain, Greece, and ancient Celtic territories. These territories also traded salt and salted foods, such as fish and fish eggs, olives, cured meats, eggs, and pickled vegetables, to various regions around the world, a trade that's been occurring for thousands of years. Almost every important Roman city was located near a source of salt, and the average Roman consumed 25 grams of salt, equivalent to 10 grams

(10,000 milligrams) of sodium per day, more than 2.5 times our current average intake.[4]

In ancient times, humans invented creative methods of salt production. They drilled brine wells in the earth and boiled the brine down to salt crystals. They extracted salt deposits from dried river-beds. They actively evaporated seawater from human-made lakes and ponds, mined mountain salt, and extracted salt from the soil in the desert or the burned ashes of marsh plants. Or they simply boiled marsh water and peat.

Before refrigeration, salt was the main antimicrobial and preservative agent, helping to maintain the freshness of foods for weeks or even months when canned properly. Salt was considered so valuable that it was used to pay Roman soldiers and was a symbol of a binding agreement. In fact, the absence of salt on a Roman dinner table was interpreted as an unfriendly act, raising suspicion. It was the life force of the ancient world.[5]

By the sixteenth century, Europeans were estimated to consume around 40 grams of salt per day; in the eighteenth century, their intake was up to 70 grams, mainly from salted cod and herring,[6] an amount four to seven times the current intake of salt in the Western world. In France, in 1725, where detailed records were kept regarding salt revenue because of heavy taxation, the daily salt intake was between 13 and 15 grams per day.[7] In Zurich, Switzerland, it was over 23 grams. Salt was consumed in even higher quantities in Scandinavian countries: consumption levels topped 50 grams of salt in Denmark, and Nils Alwall even estimated that in the sixteenth century, daily consumption of salt in Sweden *approached 100 grams* (again, mainly from salted fish and cured meat).[8]

All of this suggests that the consumption of salt throughout Europe during the last several hundred years was likely at least twice, and even up to ten times, what it is today. Now let's look at the rise of chronic disease in Europe. And how did our hearts fare during this heyday of unbridled salt consumption?

We can't be entirely sure of the prevalence of hypertension in

Europe in the 1500s to the 1800s—the blood pressure cuff was not in-vented until the late 1800s, after all—but we do know that the preva-lence of hypertension in the early 1900s in the United States was estimated at 5 to 10 percent of the population.[9] In 1939, in Chicago, the prevalence of hypertension in adults was just 11 to 13 percent. That figure then doubled to 25 percent by 1975, before finally reach-ing 31 percent in 2004.[10] This figure has continued to edge upward, and as of 2014, one out of every three adults in the United States has hypertension.[11]

Stepping back from this data, we can generalize and say that the prevalence of hypertension in the United States in the first half of the 1900s was around 10 percent. However, the prevalence of hy-pertension is now *three times as high*[12]—despite salt intake remaining remarkably stable over the last fifty years.[13]

Clearly, our salt intake did *not* parallel the rise in the prevalence of hypertension in the United States during the last half of the twen-tieth century. But what about heart disease?

We already know that salt intake was extremely high in Europe during the 1500s, somewhere between 40 and 100 grams of salt per day. If salt caused heart disease—chest pain leading to sudden death—and Europeans were consuming around 40 grams of salt per day in the 1500s,[14] there should have been *hundreds of thousands* of reports of heart disease during this time. Yet the first report did not occur until the mid-1600s.[15] And the rates of heart disease only jumped to critical levels in the early 1900s. The rise of chronic dis-ease simply does not parallel the rise of salt consumption—if any-thing, it's inversely proportional.

So how did the current nutrition guidelines come to be? Research missteps, arrogance, funding conflicts, a stubborn refusal to relent—all these forces combined together to form them and keep them in place, even today.

An Idea as Old as It Is Inaccurate

The theory that salt raises blood pressure is over one hundred years old. Two French scientists named Ambard and Beauchard are credited for inventing the salt–blood pressure hypothesis in 1904 based on findings from just six of their patients.[16] When these scientists gave these patients more salt, their blood pressure tended to go up. However, just a few years later, in 1907, Lowenstein published conflicting findings in patients with nephritis (inflammation of the kidneys).[17] For close to the next century, scientists would tussle over the relative benefits and risks of salt consumption—although the quality of the research on both sides was far from equivalent.

The Salt Wars saga first spilled over into the United States in the early 1920s. Frederick M. Allen, a medical doctor from New York, and coworkers were the first to bring salt restriction to the attention of the American medical profession as a potential therapeutic strategy for lowering blood pressure. They published four papers, two in 1920 and two in 1922, that apparently set off the controversy in the United States. The core of these papers alleged that salt restriction lowered blood pressure in around 60 percent of those with hypertension. Allen used these case reports to champion salt restriction as a potential treatment for hypertension. Going further, he hypothesized that dietary salt irritated the kidneys, overworking them and eventually leading to elevations in blood pressure even in those who still had normal kidney function. But Allen had no proof. However, his rationale seemed sound; salt restriction was said to "spare the kidney, mainly by limiting the intake of salt."[18] However, numerous publications during this time refuted the idea that salt restriction was a good option for treating hypertension, and the idea fell out of favor.[19] Over twenty years later, the "overworked kidney" theory of hypertension was plucked from obscurity and seemingly stolen by Walter Kempner, a researcher destined to create his legacy on this fallacy. Indeed, Kempner was stern in prescribing severe dietary restriction in order to relieve the kidneys of an increased workload, and this included salt restriction. He wrote, "There must be total war. Attacking one factor is not enough. Reducing the sodium is not enough; reducing cholesterol is not enough; reducing fluid and amino acids is not enough. Simple reduction is not enough, for all factors of renal work must be reduced to an absolute minimum."[20] Kempner would go on to receive worldwide recognition for the results he claimed to get with his Rice Diet—which just happened to be low in salt (one factor of about a dozen other dietary restrictions). The extrapolation of Kempner's work as proof that low-salt diets are effective for treating hypertension is one of the most egregious instances of research misinterpretation in the entire Salt Wars saga.[21]

The Kempner Rice Diet

The third child of Walter Kempner Sr. and Lydia Rabinowitsch-Kempner, Walter Kempner[22] was raised in pre–World War I Berlin, where he studied medicine, eventually graduating from the University of Heidelberg. Kempner arrived in America as a refugee from the Nazis and through good fortune began to work at Duke University. It was there that Kempner invented his infamous Rice Diet in 1939.[23]

Dr. Kempner treated hundreds of patients with his Rice Diet, compiling a large number of case reports. His analysis of his case reports suggested that a low-salt diet, consisting mainly of rice and fruit, was effective in treating most of his patients who had malignant hypertension, chronic kidney disease, and even diabetes.[24] Kempner believed that salt was a "waste product" of the kidneys, and by reducing salt, one could protect the kidneys from being overworked.[25]

The guidelines of Kempner's Rice Diet might send a shiver down the spine of any modern endocrinologist. The diet consisted of no more than 2,000 calories, 5 grams of fat, 20 grams of protein, 200 milligrams of chloride, and 150 milligrams of sodium (about $1/15$ teaspoon).[26] Rice of any kind was allowed, at an average intake of 9 to 12 ounces per day. All kinds of fruit juices and fruits were allowed with apparently no limit on their intake, but Kempner forbade the consumption of nuts, dates, avocados, canned or dried fruit, or fruit derivatives, and only the addition of white sugar was allowed. (Because we all know how much nutrition white sugar adds.)

On average, his diet contained around 100 grams of a combination of white sugar and dextrose per day—but up to 500 grams "if necessary." (Try to imagine what could possibly make 125 teaspoons of added sugar per day "necessary.") Vegetable juices or tomato juices were not allowed, and no water was given in the diet, with the fluid intake being limited to 700 to 1,000 milliliters of fruit juice per day. Once the Rice Diet was effective and conditions improved, "small amounts of non-leguminous vegetables, potatoes, lean meat or fish (all prepared without salt or fat) may be added."[27]

Kempner's case reports gained substantial media attention.[28] However, to say that his case reports were of suspect quality would be a tremendous understatement. First of all, they were not clinical trials, so he could not prove causation. Kempner did not have a control group with whom to compare his patients, nor did he use adequate control periods after hospitalization. The flaws in his research meant that his results could have been completely spurious findings, having nothing to do with the diet. In fact, one of the most likely reasons for the diet's "success" was his somewhat idiosyncratic style of monitoring his patients: Kempner was said to watch his patients "like a hawk"[29]—he even admitted to *whipping* his patients who strayed from the diet.[30]

Even back then, fellow researchers questioned whether the low-salt aspect of his Rice Diet was the reason for its effectiveness. Indeed, one of Kempner's own patients with hypertension, ascites, and edema found that all three conditions were unchanged after following a standard low-salt diet. The patient's blood pressure was 174/97 mmHg, but approximately two months after being placed on the Rice Diet, his blood pressure dropped to 137/82 mmHg—not surprisingly, a change that coincided with a 14-kilogram weight loss.[31]

The Rice Diet was found to dangerously deplete salt in the body, drastically lowering plasma chloride from 97 mEq/L to 91.7 mEq/L.[32]

(Bear in mind that chloride levels lower than 100 mEq/L are independently associated with higher mortality.[33]) According to Kempner himself, the Rice Diet was ineffective at significantly lowering blood pressure in 178 of 500 patients (about 36 percent). But he focused his claims exclusively on the 322 of 500 patients (about 64 percent) in whom the diet decreased mean arterial blood pressure by at least 20 mmHg.[34] Even if we can consider these results true, they could have been due to one of any number of factors from the Rice Diet that had little to do with salt restriction: the increase in the intake of potassium and fiber; the reduction in protein, fat, trans fat, and seed oils; and the overall reduction in caloric intake and, hence, weight loss. Yet those facets of the diet were rarely factored into the explanation of its results.

Regardless of the fact that not everyone benefited from the diet—again, a full third did not—Kempner's low-salt Rice Diet was thereafter generally recognized as being an effective therapy and is still cited, even today, as proof that low-salt diets are effective for treating hypertension, kidney disease, and heart failure.

Another detail that was rarely mentioned in the lionizing of Kempner's evidence was one cogent fact: Kempner's patients had all been extremely sick at the start of their treatment. They had an average baseline blood pressure of 199/117 mmHg, which is considered hypertensive crisis.[35] This fact alone should have disqualified the Rice Diet's presumed effectiveness for the general public.[36] And, sure enough—and not surprisingly—when others tested the Rice Diet, the results were far less convincing than what Kempner was finding.

In one study of patients with essential hypertension who tried a version of the Rice Diet, 83 percent were found to have no reduction in blood pressure.[37] Of the ten patients whose kidney function was measured, nine had a reduced glomerular filtration rate, a marker of kidney function; eight had reduced renal blood flow; and in six, the maximal tubular excretory capacity was reduced. In other words, the low-salt, low-protein diet in patients with essential hypertension seemed to *worsen* kidney function and was ineffective at treating high blood pressure.

This was the opposite of what Kempner was reporting.

More troubling was a Medical Research Council (MRC) report, published in the *Lancet* in 1950, indicating that a patient had died of uremia (excess urea, or urine, in the blood due to kidney disease) on the low-salt Rice Diet.[38] The authors argued that a kidney already damaged by hypertension might be less able to reabsorb salt, dangerously lowering the salt levels in the blood, and that those with renal failure might be tremendously harmed by reducing salt.

Trials continued to poke holes in Kempner's findings, and in 1983, John Laragh, renowned founder of the Hypertension Center at New York–Presbyterian/Weill Cornell Medical Center, and colleagues published a review paper citing those who had performed better-controlled studies and had reported less-beneficial results. They found that the diet was only effective in 20 to 40 percent of patients, compared to Kempner's claim of 64 percent effectiveness.[39] Also, when researchers tried to tease out the beneficial components of the diet, they found that salt restriction (generally less than 1.15 grams per day) seemed to *reverse* the benefits of the Rice Diet.[40] So the primary claim about the diet was, in fact, the thing that made it *less* effective. With the benefit of hindsight, if we can take away anything from Kempner's Rice Diet, it's that we should increase our intake of potassium and fiber in the form of fruit and whole grains—that alone may do the trick.

At this point, almost thirty-five years ago, Laragh and colleagues suggested that there was no evidence that moderate salt restriction would prevent hypertension on a population-wide scale,[41] and even in those who are considered "salt-sensitive"—those 25 to 45 percent in whom salt restriction does slightly reduce blood pressure—there was only weak evidence that it worked. Laragh and colleagues concluded that the weight loss and reduction in blood pressure with the Rice Diet was actually entirely independent of salt intake.[42] They went on to suggest that only for those in whom sodium restriction had been proven to be "effective" should salt reduction be implemented.

Still others tested the low-salt diet and found it lacking. Arthur Corcoran and his colleagues at Cleveland Clinic Research Division (which Corcoran established) showed that even in patients with "severe essential hypertension," a low-salt diet only provided benefit in about 25 percent. In contrast, definite *harms* were noted, such as azotemia (a high level of urea, creatinine, and other nitrogen-rich waste in the blood) and worsening kidney function. They found that most people had to get their daily sodium intake all the way down to just 200 milligrams *or less* (the equivalent of less than $1/11$ teaspoon of salt) in order to get a reduction in blood pressure, which was completely impractical if not impossible.[43]

Indeed, in all of the studies done on the diet, only 28 percent of those who attempted it could even adhere to the Rice Diet, and only 37 percent of those who adhered to the Rice Diet showed an improvement in blood pressure. Whenever Kempner tested his "method," 62 percent of patients experienced an improvement in blood pressure.[44] (Presumably after being beaten into compliance!) But curiously, no other researcher could duplicate this finding, and when tested by others, the Rice Diet was found to cause harm.

The known consequences of salt restriction, such as low sodium and chloride in the blood, have long been independently known to increase the risk of death.[45] And azotemia, kidney failure, and even several deaths have occurred on the low-salt Rice Diet.[46] Other side effects reported include lack of energy, anorexia, nausea, abnormally small amounts of urine production (oliguria), muscle twitching and abdominal cramps, and uremia (urea buildup in the blood), likely indicating kidney failure. Unfortunately, both during Kempner's time and even today, the serious risks of low-salt diets are rarely, if ever, mentioned in any guidelines recommending them, despite the pleas of many researchers about the weakness of the salt–blood pressure hypothesis. "The assumption that only moderate sodium deprivation would accomplish [decreased risk of hypertension in the general population] is even greater speculation. Furthermore, the idea that moderate reduction in dietary salt throughout our society would be harmless is unproved," said Schroeder and Goldman, in a piece published in the *Journal of the American Medical Association* (JAMA) in 1949.[47] Many researchers remained skeptical about recommending blanket salt reduction to the general public, and over the next several decades, others had reported much less effectiveness of Kempner's Rice Diet (and low-salt diets in general); salt restriction as a means to prevent and treat hypertension generally fell out of favor.

That is, until Lewis K. Dahl.

Lewis K. Dahl

Dr. Lewis Kitchener Dahl was said to be a man of "strong conviction."[48] Dahl originally took an interest in the notion that certain populations who (apparently) consumed a low-salt diet did not have much hypertension, such as the Inuit. In contrast, those who consumed high amounts of salt, such as the Japanese, had a much higher rate of hypertension.[49] This led him to study the effects of salt in rodents. However, there was a problem: Dahl knew that salt didn't have much effect on blood pressure in normal rats. So he decided to selectively modify them through inbreeding over several generations in order to create what is now known as "Dahl salt-sensitive rats." That's right: Dahl *created* salt-sensitive rats in a lab, and then used them to prove his salt–blood pressure hypothesis.[50]

In 1954, Lewis K. Dahl and Robert A. Love from the Medical Research Center, Brookhaven National Laboratory, Upton, New York, published a paper in the American Medical Association's *Archives of Internal Medicine* that was later credited with reviving the idea that a high-sodium diet was driving the high prevalence of hypertension in the Western world.[51] Primarily basing their assertions on epidemiological studies, Dahl and Love cited evidence that primitive societies who ate a low-salt diet were leaner, were more active, and didn't develop high blood pressure—without acknowledging that these same societies seldom ate a high-sugar diet, either. For some reason, the idea that obesity itself could lead to hypertension (and that both could be driven by sugar) was not a popular theory at the time. The fact that there wasn't a single publication until 1983 showing that sugar raises blood pressure in humans didn't help matters.[52] (And lest we cast stones at those researchers of yore and consider them myopic, acknowledge the fact that even today we generally don't tend to think that one disease could be related to another. We like to separate diseases from one another and treat each disease via different specialists—but that's clearly not how the body actually works.)

By the mid-1950s, despite many experts lobbying to the contrary, salt had already been demonized as the blood pressure–raising white crystal. To make matters worse, the sugar industry was working hard to help shift the blame off sugar and over to other dietary substances (like saturated fat).[53] And this blame-shifting would also leave salt out to dry as the white crystal that causes hypertension—no one was even considering sugar. Why would they? At the time, sugar was considered completely harmless by most scientists, and certainly by most of the lay public.

Dahl was then one of the first to propose that added salt is a condiment—not a dietary need. In 1960, he published a review of the literature from studies he had gathered since 1954,[54] showing that in five populations, as the intake of salt increased, so did the prevalence of hypertension. He even went so far as to conclude that humans could easily *survive* on less than 1 gram of salt per day. He cited some of his own studies in which the intake of salt was apparently dropped to around 100 to 375 milligrams per day, sustained for three to twelve months. He also referenced three people who'd apparently had a "proven" intake of salt between 250 and 375 milligrams for two to five years, and how a seventeen-year-old girl was able to "maintain salt balance" on an intake of just 10 to 12 milligrams of salt for several months (but no reference was provided for the latter).[55] Despite all of this "evidence," none of the work Dahl presented truly proved that low-salt diets were beneficial or without harm.

Dahl cited evidence that giving salt to rats that were genetically engineered to be *susceptible* to salt produced hypertension—without mentioning the equivalent human dose of salt in these studies. According to Bjorn Folkow, esteemed author of over four hundred articles on vascular physiology and a member of the Royal Swedish Academy of Sciences, that human equivalent would have been 40 grams of salt per day (or over four times a normal salt intake). That's how much salt it would take to raise blood pressure in similarly salt-sensitive humans.[56] In the salt-resistant rats—those that didn't have a blood pressure "problem" with salt—even the human equivalent of 100 grams of salt per day *still* did not raise the blood pressure.

It's safe to say that the rat studies cited by Lewis Dahl were completely irrelevant to humans. But Dahl was undeterred. To buttress his case, Dahl cited a 1945 JAMA publication as proof that low-salt diets lowered blood pressure in humans. One problem: that publication did not in any way show that salt restriction lowered blood pressure significantly in everyone. In fact, a closer look at that paper suggests the low-salt study may have actually *killed* people.[57] One patient who was placed on the low-salt diet died soon afterward; another sustained circulatory collapse, which usually suggests a failure to maintain a supply of oxygen and nutrients to the tissues. When salt was added back into the diet, the patient with circulatory collapse improved (thank goodness).

These important points were not mentioned by Dahl in his paper. And yet Dahl was so convinced that salt causes hypertension, he concluded, "This idea [that salt causes hypertension] is today so widely accepted and used that dilation would belabor the obvious." But perhaps it would have been instructive to have a bit more "obvious dilation" before pinning public health policy to this flawed theory for several more decades.

Dahl even suggested that the high salt level in infant foods was to blame for the high infant mortality rate in the United States.[58] When he gave certain baby formulas to salt-sensitive rats, they would end up dead. But of course human babies are much larger than rats, and salt-sensitive rats aren't normal rats—but Dahl didn't let that stop him. He issued a blanket proclamation that salt in baby formulas could be harmful to infants. Never mind that in his experiments, these salt-sensitive rats were developing malignant hypertension, which was leading to their death[59]—something that was not occurring in human babies. Based partly on Dahl's work and ideas, the Committee on Nutrition of the American Academy of Pediatrics concluded that salt intake of infants was too high, and manufacturers began to lower the salt content of their foods.[60]

Quality in research counts—but somehow, throughout the Salt Wars, the power of sheer personal stubbornness and a hesitancy to question the status quo overwhelmed the power of academic rigor and integrity. And we've been paying the price ever since.

George Meneely and Harold Battarbee

Two authors likely had the greatest influence for getting salt restriction integrated into the 1977 Dietary Goals: George R. Meneely and Harold D. Battarbee from Louisiana State University Medical Center were among the most renowned scientists supporting the notion that salt restriction helps prevent and treat high blood pressure.[61] Indeed, Meneely was actually the head of the physiology and biophysics department at Louisiana State, a position that afforded him a lot of clout and admiration.[62] Both Meneely and Battarbee believed that a high-sodium/low-potassium diet was the principal driver of hypertension.[63] They wrote that "excess salt" leads to expansion of the extracellular fluid volume and increased blood pressure—but they never specifically stated *what* amount of salt causes these consequences.

Even Meneely and Battarbee acknowledged that the idea that salt causes hypertension was just a theory in their 1976 paper titled "High Sodium-Low Potassium Environment and Hypertension." Their paper was one of the most comprehensive reviews looking at salt and blood pressure at the time, and it was published just prior to the 1977 Dietary Goals. All this gave these authors a lot of notoriety. And the fact that the salt–blood pressure connection was just a theory got lost in the fanfare—and one can imagine, given the attention the authors were receiving, that they preferred not to soften the impact of their work. In fact, in the U.S. Senate report, Meneely and Battarbee were quoted in the Senate Report's Supplementary Views, having testified before the Senate Committee in support of salt restriction.[64]

What wasn't given much attention by the U.S. Senate or the 1977 Dietary Goals, however, was that their theory was a *combination* of a *high-salt* and *low-potassium* intake that leads to hypertension, and still only in those who were *genetically susceptible*. These details were overshadowed by the big headline: salt leads to hypertension. But this little blip of coincidental timing turned out to have monumental impact on our nation's health for the next forty years. The public was told that *everyone* would benefit from salt restriction and that it was a safe intervention to prevent and treat hypertension—something the evidence in the literature had never supported, before or since.

In 1977, George McGovern's Senate Select Committee on Nutrition and Human Needs published the Dietary Goals, which recommended that all Americans restrict their salt intake to just 3 grams (1.2 grams of sodium) per day.[65] This guideline was based on expert opinion at the time rather than sound evidence. Indeed, during this time, sound evidence was not a requirement to give dietary guidance to the nation; there was no demand for systematic reviews of the literature, or even evidence from clinical trials in humans. If you were considered an expert and had enough clout, your word would be considered "evidence." A massive public health dictum that radically impacted food policy, industry regulations, school lunch programs, and physicians' standard of care for subsequent decades was, in essence, based on the opinions of just a few scientists (and nonscientists, for that matter).

After the Dietary Goals were published in February 1977, two other hearings occurred to address around fifty additional opinions. These hearings were held on March 24 and July 26, and notes of these hearings were published in the Supplemental Views. These Supplemental Views offer a glimpse into the origin of the severe limits on salt intake: The Senate Select Committee relied mostly on the National Academy of Sciences (a nonprofit organization composed of the nation's leading researchers) and George Meneely and Harold Battarbee for recommending a limit of just 3 grams of salt per day.[66] We can thank Meneely and Battarbee for at least contributing to the 3-grams-per-day salt limit given to all Americans.[67]

By the time the second edition of the 1977 Dietary Goals was published, less than one year later, the limit of 3 grams of salt per day had been increased to 5 grams (around 2 grams of sodium). This might have been due to additional testimony provided to the Senate Select Committee indicating that even if someone obtained an entire 3 grams of salt as the iodized form, they still would not achieve the recommended amount of iodine per day (150 micrograms).[68] (Even today, the populations of fifty-four countries are still considered iodine deficient, and our best way of obtaining iodine is—you guessed it—by eating iodized salt.)[69] Again, the emphasis was on the minimum necessary to preserve life—hardly a metric for vital health.

The Supplemental Views reflected a robust dialogue about salt guidelines. They also referred to consumer warnings about salt restriction for people on medications that eliminate salt or lead to salt depletion. And even the American Heart Association was quoted as stating that "with the advent of effective sodium-eliminating diuretics, *the need for strongly-restricted sodium diets has been sharply modified* [emphasis added]." The American Medical Association (AMA) stated, "While epidemiological observations suggest a relation between salt ingestion and hypertension, *they fail to support the hypothesis that salt consumption is a major factor in causing hypertension in persons in the United States* [emphasis added]." And the Committee on Nutrition of the American Academy of Pediatrics stated, "The role of salt intake as an environmental factor in the induction of hypertension has still to be defined. *For 80 percent of the population in this country, present salt intake has not been demonstrated to be harmful, i.e., hypertension has not developed* [emphasis added]." In other words, three major medical establishments were wary of the low-salt advice given to all Americans at the very outset of the 1977 Dietary Goals.

REVERSING THE DANGERS OF DIURETICS

A few years ago, I was counseling a woman in her mid-forties who had been feeling light-headed and claimed to be "always craving salt." She had high blood pressure and had been put on a salt-excreting diuretic called hydrochlorothiazide, and was adamantly told by her doctor to not salt her foods and to avoid salt in her diet. However, I was concerned that her light-headedness and salt cravings were a signal, that her body was telling her something was wrong.

I told her she should get her blood sodium level drawn to make sure it was normal (usually around 137–142 mEq/L). She called the pharmacy and asked to speak to me and told me that her blood sodium level at the doctor's office was just 128 mEq/L. (To put this number in perspective: a blood sodium level of 125 mEq/L can be fatal.) Based on her diagnosis of hyponatremia (low sodium in the blood), the doctor cut her diuretic dose in half. He also told her I was right: she *should* consume salt when she had a salt craving.

A few weeks after her diuretic dose had been cut in half and she'd been consuming salt when her body told her she needed it, her blood sodium level was back to virtually normal (136 mEq/L). This is a perfect example of why we should not blindly follow the advice from "well-meaning" dietary guidelines and health agencies. Real-world situations cannot be encapsulated into "guidelines."

Had these distinguished organizations pressed their case, rather than allow the flawed work of several individuals to represent the entire medical community, we might have never been asked to give up the saltshaker. Our health, and in particular our quality of life, might not have needed to suffer. But the Salt Wars were destined to rage on for another forty years, all the way up to today.

Formally Enshrining the Low-Salt Guidelines

Throughout the Salt Wars, studies consistently contradicted each other, the findings bouncing back and forth like a never-ending tennis match. Some studies showed that salt increased blood pressure,[70] but others did not.[71] The supporters of the salt–blood pressure hypothesis continually argued that the skeptics had little merit—and there were many advocates of the salt–blood pressure hypothesis.

Arthur Guyton, an American physiologist, was one of the most influential voices in the early 1980s. He believed that an increase in extracellular fluid from increased salt intake could lead to hypertension.[72] However, he also believed that the kidneys would have to be compromised in order for this to occur, as it was well known that any extra salt in the body can easily be excreted by the kidneys.[73] What was harming the kidneys and creating "salt-sensitive hypertension," however, was not known at the time. (Spoiler alert: it's the other white crystal.)[74]

While some studies looking *across* populations found an association between salt consumption and blood pressure, this same effect could not be found when looking *within* populations. Meneely and Battarbee argued for a "saturation effect," saying that when an entire population eats an excessive amount of salt, any evidence that could correlate salt intake with blood pressure would be hidden—when these effects were actually more likely attributable to lower potassium intake and higher consumption of sugar and refined carbohydrate.[75] And this rationale seemed to work—but even the low-salt advocates found it hard to make a case for salt restriction. Only one out of four people is able to comply with rigid salt restriction, making it a rather futile public health policy.[76]

Despite the average person's struggles to comply, Lewis Dahl was having none of it. He and other low-salt advocates simply demanded that the public needed to work harder to curb their salt appetite.[77]

In 1983, six years after the publication of the 1977 Dietary Goals, founder of the Hypertension Center at New York-Presbyterian/Weill Cornell Medical Center John Laragh[78] and colleagues published a paper that exposed some of the misguided leaps, perpetuated by the low-salt advocates, that had led the country to adopting such stringent guidelines. Laragh and company alleged that, all told, fewer than two hundred patients had ever been tested with moderate salt restriction to treat hypertension.[79] Laragh also stressed that most of the studies were of short duration and they didn't look at hard endpoints (such as cardiovascular events or death). Despite these poor-quality results, every American had been told to restrict their salt intake by sweeping public health mandates. Additionally, no clear benefits had been found in those with normal blood pressure who restricted salt. The "benefits" of low-salt diets in patients with hypertension (again, based only on a few hundred patients) had been extrapolated to everyone in the United States, even those with normal blood pressure.

One of the best studies of the time was conducted in 1982, when British cardiovascular researcher Graham MacGregor and colleagues at Charing Cross Medical School in London tested just nineteen patients with mild to moderate essential hypertension in a placebo-controlled trial. The crossover trial tested a low-salt diet (1,840 milligrams of sodium per day) and a normal-salt diet (3,680 milligrams of sodium per day).[80] While the average blood pressure was around 9/5 mmHg lower on the low-salt diet, some of the nineteen patients apparently had no significant benefit, and two patients actually experienced slight increases in blood pressure with salt restriction. Importantly, based on twenty-four-hour urinary potassium levels, the intake of potassium in the trial was low (around 2.2 to 2.5 grams per day, or about half the recommended intake of 4.7 grams of potassium per day[81]). What this trial actually showed was that compared to a normal-salt diet combined with a low potassium intake, a low-salt diet lowers blood pressure in some hypertensive patients but may raise blood pressure in others. In other words, mixed results. This study exemplifies the problems of extrapolating results from controlled clinical settings to the outside world. No one considered that adding salt to vegetables would increase our liking for them and hence how much of them we consume. In other words, using salt allows us to consume more vegetables (i.e., potassium), which leads to an overall improvement in our health and blood pressure. Instead, we were being given the wrong message based on evidence that had little to do with how people actually live.

Sadly, MacGregor chose to stick with the flawed interpretation of these results and took up the mission of salt reduction on a global scale. After this study, MacGregor began his unrelenting one-man crusade against salt that has continued for decades and has positioned him on governmental and health agency advisory boards, wielding his influence widely. He's been extremely effective in shaming industries and public health agencies into bending to his will.

MacGregor started Consensus Action on Salt and Health (CASH) in 1995[82] and followed up by creating World Action on Salt and Health (WASH) in 2005.[83] With these two anti-salt research and advocacy groups, MacGregor had an elevated platform from which to spread his fervent belief that salt raises blood pressure and thus *must* raise the risk of stroke and heart attacks. Secure in that belief, he has been lobbying governments around the world relentlessly for decades to lower salt intake and the salt content of foods. In fact, CASH has been very successful and influential in getting UK food manufacturers to lower their salt content, despite the lack of research backing, and as many as eighty other countries are considering adopting the same guidelines MacGregor forced through in the UK. One reason his efforts may have been more persuasive is that he has lumped salt with other food additives—such as unhealthy fats and added sugar—which both boast much more plausible data showing negative health outcomes.

MacGregor has been emphatic about the evils of salt, his focus trained solely on the supposed benefits to lowered blood pressure as protection against heart disease. Meanwhile, these groups (CASH and WASH) simply dismissed the harms of low-salt diets. When small reductions in blood pressure were placed into "risk calculators," these groups would shout from the rooftops about the benefits of low-salt diets. The harms of low-salt, however, were never inserted in these calculators. Not surprisingly, they always concluded that "lowering salt will save lives" based only on reductions in blood pressure, but never by computing the harms of the higher heart rate, triglycerides, cholesterol, and insulin levels—all factors with much more thoroughly and rigorously documented links to heart disease. CASH and WASH have continued to promote that unproven direct link—that low-salt saves lives—for decades.[84]

Once an idea is entrenched in people's minds, it is hard to supplant it. And the research to the contrary hadn't been adequately translated and presented to the American public. Even the Dietary Guidelines for Americans, first published in 1980, have continued to tell Americans to cut back on their salt intake. Limited expert opinion turned into established public health policy, and health policy became unassailable low-salt dogma.

The first systematic review of trials testing the low-salt advice wasn't published until 1991, almost fifteen years after the 1977 Dietary Goals told us to restrict our salt intake. This systematic review, performed by Law and colleagues, included seventy-eight trials, only ten of which were randomized.[85] This systematic review became the basis for why the U.S. hypertension guidelines promoted low-salt diets in the general public, as it contended that a reduction of 2,300 milligrams per day of sodium would drop blood pressure by 10/5 mmHg in people with normal blood pressure and 14/7 mmHg in people with hypertension. Law and colleagues went on to state that low-salt diets could prevent seventy thousand deaths per year in Britain (based solely on the potential reduction in blood pressure). These strong statements were clearly aimed to unite a group worn down by the Salt Wars controversy.

However, these benefits on blood pressure were significantly greater than results found a few years later from higher-quality meta-analyses that included only randomized data. For example, in people with normal blood pressure, the newer, stronger meta-analyses of salt-restriction trials reported *one-tenth* the impact on systolic pressure and *one-fiftieth* the impact on diastolic pressure compared to the analysis by Law and colleagues (−1/0.1 mmHg compared to −10/5 mmHg).[86] Despite all of this higher-quality evidence showing that this reduction made only an inconsequential impact, in 1993 the Hypertension Guidelines in the United States (the Joint National Committee on Detection, Evaluation, and Treatment of High Blood Pressure [JNC 5])[87] decided to cite the earlier Law meta-analysis to conclude that a modest reduction in the intake of sodium (1,150 milligrams of sodium) would reduce systolic blood pressure by 7 mmHg in people with hypertension and 5 mmHg in those with normal blood pressure.

Between 1991 and 1998, the Law 1991 meta-analysis was cited more than any other, despite being the weakest. Any findings in support of salt restriction were cited more than negative ones.[88]

Finally, a heavyweight stepped up to the plate. John D. Swales, a doctor, hypertension expert, and founding editor of the *Journal of Hypertension*, published a paper in 2000 showing that people with normal blood pressure only get a small reduction in systolic (1 to 2 mmHg) and diastolic (0.1 to 1 mmHg) blood pressure when they severely restrict their sodium intake.[89] Moreover, Swales wrote that the low-salt recommendations were based on data that had been "amplified by publication bias" (the tendency to publish positive rather than negative results); that the amount of salt restriction to obtain the small reductions in blood pressure was unachievable by the public; and that the results could be due to other changes in the diet besides just a reduction in salt. Swales also stated that there was a cost to lowering salt intake, both a social/quality-of-life cost and an economic cost. These considerations had long been looked down upon as almost irrelevant.

Swales went on to cite six meta-analyses of salt restriction in his paper, five of which contained only randomized trials and one meta-analysis that contained both randomized and nonrandomized studies. The five meta-analyses with randomized trials found that in people with normal blood pressure, salt restriction did not even reduce systolic blood pressure by 2 mmHg—not even 2 points! Only one meta-analysis of the five found a reduction in diastolic blood pressure greater than 1 mmHg—the rest were between 0.1 mmHg and 0.97 mmHg.

At best, the research suggested, salt restriction in people with normal blood pressure caused a reduction in blood pressure of only around 2/1 mmHg. Three of the meta-analyses concluded that dietary salt restriction was not supported by the evidence,[90] with only one concluding that there was "great potential" with salt restriction.[91] However, this "great potential" for salt restriction and blood pressure lowering was based on trials with a reduction in sodium intake between 1,748 milligrams and 3,680 milligrams, which is highly unlikely to occur in the general population. In fact, longer-performed sodium-restriction trials indicate that the public might be able to achieve a reduction in sodium intake of around 1,000 milligrams at the very most.[92] In other words, the "great potential" of lowering blood pressure via salt restriction was based on a reduction of salt two to three times the amount the public would likely be able to achieve.

Many low-salt advocates argued that salt-restriction trials hadn't been performed long enough to show a benefit, yet a systematic review of eight randomized controlled trials looking at salt restriction of greater than six months found similarly small reductions in systolic blood pressure (−2.9 mmHg in people with hypertension and −1.3 mmHg in people with normal blood pressure).[93] More importantly, a systematic review by Law and colleagues suggested that it took just four weeks to get the maximal reductions in blood pressure with low-salt diets, and another review of randomized trials did not find progressive blood pressure lowering over time with salt restriction.[94]

Perhaps most importantly, a meta-analysis performed by Midgley and colleagues underscored the influence of publication bias with the sodium-restriction trials. It found that trials that tested low sodium with positive results were more likely to be published compared to negative trials.[95] Midgley emphasized that publication bias had led the scientific community to overestimate the blood-pressure-lowering benefits of salt reduction. This publication bias continues to distort the Salt Wars, even to this day.

The Huge Shadow of Intersalt

In 1989, the Food and Nutrition Board's "Diet and Health: Implications for Reducing Chronic Disease Risk" set a maximum intake of 2,400 milligrams of sodium. This was based on the 1988 Intersalt study, a massive epidemiological study conducted at fifty-two population centers around the world, led by Dr. Paul Elliot from the Department of Epidemiology, London School of Hygiene and Tropical Medicine, London. The Food and Nutrition Board claimed that the Intersalt study proved that blood pressure increased with age if sodium intake was above 2,400 milligrams per day.[96] One problem: the Intersalt study showed the opposite. Only five populations of the fifty-two studied consumed less than 2,400 milligrams daily, and four of them were primitive societies. The fifth population that consumed under 2,400 milligrams of sodium actually had a higher systolic blood pressure compared to several populations with a higher salt intake. In fact, one population consumed more than twice the amount of salt but had a lower systolic blood pressure. And when the four primitive societies were excluded from the other fifty-two populations, the data shifted—suddenly there was a clear downward slope for blood pressure as salt intake increased.[97]

That's right: as salt intake increased, blood pressure actually declined. The 2,400-milligram Daily Value for sodium (printed on every Nutrition Facts label) is the perfect example of the anti-salt warriors' Napoleon complex: quick to exaggerate in order to make up for lack of evidence. There really never was good evidence for setting a limit of 2,400 milligrams of sodium per day, but this target was sealed onto every Nutrition Facts label and subsequently carried over to the 1995 Dietary Guidelines for Americans.

What is most chilling is the apparent decision by the Intersalt group not to publish data on heart rate. Heart rate was supposedly measured in the study, at least according to Bjorn Folkow, who reported that Paul Elliot (the corresponding author of Intersalt) had communicated to him that heart rate was measured in Intersalt.[98] We likely will never know why this heart rate data was never published by the Intersalt group, but it's well known that low-salt diets increase heart rate.[99] Could Intersalt be just another example of "publish findings that support your theory and bury the ones that don't"? The official line is that the Intersalt group "declined to make their underlying data public . . . because of the need to preserve the independence of scientific investigation, the integrity of the data, and the confidentiality of information."[100] This explanation by these authors seems to be without any logic.

An alternate explanation: if the heart rate data were indeed measured and published, Intersalt would have likely shown harm with low-salt diets. Indeed, as Folkow suggested, the total stress on the heart and arteries comes from a combination of blood pressure and heart rate—a fact well accepted by the medical community, except when it comes to sodium intake! Folkow concluded that low-salt diets would *increase* the overall stress on the heart and arteries and hence *increase* the risk of hypertension and heart failure.[101]

The Search for the Lowest Common Denominator

By 2005, the Institute of Medicine (IOM) determined what it believed to be an adequate intake (AI) of sodium, a minimum level at which there would be a low probability of becoming salt deficient. The sodium AI was meant to cover sodium losses through sweat, even in unacclimatized individuals, to meet the needs of both healthy and moderately active people. In those who were nine to fifty years old, the AI for sodium was listed at 1,500 milligrams per day (and even lower levels for those younger and older). However, the AI did not apply to individuals who were "highly active" or "workers exposed to extreme heat stress."[102]

But how did the IOM determine that 1,500 milligrams of sodium was an adequate intake? Apparently, that figure took two metrics into account.

1. The "benefits" of blood pressure reduction with a reduction in salt—without any attention paid to the possible harms of salt restriction (such as rises in renin, aldosterone, norepinephrine, lipids, insulin, and heart rate).
2. Salt losses via urine, skin, and feces—without factoring in salt losses from medications, lifestyles (caffeine or low-carb diets), or current disease states.[103]

The IOM also set a tolerable upper intake level (UL) for sodium at 2,300 milligrams per day for adolescents and adults of all ages (fourteen years and older). The UL is the highest daily nutrient intake level that is likely not to pose risk of adverse health effects. For sodium, the UL was based on several trials, including data from the Dietary Approaches to Stop Hypertension (DASH)-Sodium trial.[104] It was noted in the DASH-Sodium trial and other trials evaluated by the IOM that blood pressure was lowered when sodium intake was reduced to 2,300 milligrams per day, and that this level of intake was the next level above the AI of 1,500 milligrams per day. Hence, the 2,300-milligram UL on sodium was based on a surrogate marker (blood pressure), not on hard endpoints such as strokes or heart attacks.

The IOM's 2,300-milligram UL of sodium was then incorporated into the 2005 Dietary Guidelines, which recommended that all Americans restrict their sodium intake to less than 2,300 milligrams.[105] Additionally, "individuals with *hypertension, blacks, and middle-aged and older adults* [emphasis added]" were recommended to consume no more than 1,500 milligrams of sodium per day. Interestingly, 2005 was the first year that the Dietary Guidelines for Americans specifically recommended lowering salt intake to lower the *risk* of high blood pressure. Back in 1980, the Dietary Guidelines had stated that lowering salt mainly applied to people with high blood pressure ("the major hazard of excessive sodium is for persons who have high blood pressure"). How did that happen?

It may have been the influence of Lawrence Appel, MD.[106] Appel was not only chair of the 2005 Institute of Medicine Panel on Dietary Reference intakes for electrolytes and water[107] and a spokesperson for the American Heart Association—he was also on the board of WASH,[108] a group whose stated purpose was to reduce sodium intake around the world. Appel had long focused only on blood pressure as a surrogate marker, translating that "benefit" on blood pressure with low salt intakes to definitive reductions in strokes and heart attacks. Like all low-salt advocates, Appel continued to ignore the harmful effects caused by sodium restriction on numerous other measures of health (called surrogate markers) such as increases in renin, aldosterone, triglycerides, cholesterol, LDL, insulin, and heart rate.

Despite his potential bias and conflict of interest as part of a group whose sole focus is to reduce sodium intake around the globe, Appel was also appointed as a member of the 2005 and 2010 Dietary Guidelines Advisory Committee. Sure enough, the Dietary Guidelines for Americans followed the IOM (of which Appel was chair regarding the recommendations for sodium intakes in the first place) and began specifically recommending low sodium intake for Americans. Indeed, those 2010 Dietary Guidelines for Americans were the first to recommend that 1,500 milligrams of sodium should be the goal for about half the U.S. population (including children and most adults). This applied to "persons who are 51 and older and those of any age who are African American or have hypertension, diabetes, or chronic kidney disease."[109] While the 1,500-milligram sodium-restriction level was removed from the 2015 Dietary Guidelines for Americans recommendations, the 2,300-milligram level remains. Finally, we begin to see a bit of nuance in the guidelines. What had previously felt like a sledgehammer in search of a fly to smash, now began to hint at what we in the field have known for decades: low salt only works for a very small subgroup of people.

And at this point, we finally—*finally*—started seeing public health leaders begin to place more emphasis on the quiet killer that had been stalking us all along, damaging our kidneys (and, indeed, *creating* our issues with salt), generally laying waste to our overall health. The white crystal that was truly deserving of the "toxic" mantle: sugar.

Sugar's Free Pass

Beginning in the 1950s, an American scientist named Ancel Keys was promoting the idea that dietary fat (and eventually saturated fat) was the cause of heart disease. At the same time, England's John Yudkin thought the blame rested with sugar.[110] But in 1961, the American Heart Association (AHA) officially demonized saturated fat, suggesting that Americans reduce their intake of animal fat and increase their intake of vegetable oils to reduce the risk of heart disease.[111] Once the AHA had officially backed the fat-heart hypothesis—that saturated fat increased cholesterol levels and, thereby, the risk for heart disease—sugar was exonerated by omission. This black-or-white, one-or-the-other choice, made on behalf of the nation, was a major reason other researchers continued to struggle to be taken seriously when they suggested sugar was a driver of heart disease. In contrast, salt wasn't exonerated, it was attacked, convicted of being an "unnecessary evil" by the National High Blood Pressure Education Program as early as 1972.[112]

So, for years, sugar was a bit like Switzerland—neutral—and it was given a free pass on the dietary front. While salt (and fat) were viewed as harmful, sugar was considered *harmless*, no better or worse for you than any other food ingredient, as long as you burned more sugar calories than you took in.

This viewpoint was vigorously perpetuated by the Sugar Association, which has engaged in strong lobbying of Congress, the Department of Health and Human Services, and various health organizations to allow sugar to maintain its benign status for many years.[113] The sugar industry has also worked hard to achieve a positive public image by sponsoring high-profile events such as the Olympics and investing in tooth decay prevention campaigns, and generally, relentlessly, shifting the focus of public health policy away from sugar.[114] It even funded scientists who seemed to downplay the harms of sugar and who were placing the blame of our increasing waistlines on a lack of exercise rather than an overconsumption of sugar.[115]

In 1977, the sugar industry was citing Jean Mayer, a professor at the Harvard School of Public Health, who suggested that the obesity problem in modern societies was caused by inactivity. By shifting the focus of obesity away from "harmful calories" and toward "total calories," sugar was able to fly under the radar of close scientific scrutiny. And because saturated fat contained more calories per gram than sugar, it took center stage as a driver of obesity, too.[116]

In 1975, just a few years prior to the publication of the 1977 Dietary Goals, Alexander R. Walker published a paper suggesting that sugar was not a cause of hypertension or heart disease. He cited three of his own studies supporting this idea; all three were apparently funded in part by the sugar industry.[117] This cozy relationship has been a common theme throughout history, in which authors who have conflicts of interest with the sugar industry consistently suggest that sugar is not inherently harmful,[118] whereas authors without conflicts of interest with the industry generally report the opposite.[119]

Strangely enough, the first edition of the 1977 Dietary Goals did recommend that we limit our consumption of added sugars to just 15 percent of our total calories,[120] and the second edition trimmed this down further, to just 10 percent of our total caloric intake, for refined and processed sugars.[121] Oh, how many lives might we have saved if that recommendation had resonated more loudly! However, over the subsequent years, the media mainly focused on salt (which hit the cover of TIME in 1982[122]), cholesterol (TIME, 1984[123]), and saturated fat (which had already hit TIME magazine in 1961[124]), and no one was taking the limits on the intake of sugar seriously. Indeed, over the next twenty years, from 1980 until 2000,[125] the Dietary Guidelines for Americans told us that sugar did not cause diabetes or heart disease, despite clear evidence to the contrary.[126]

In 1979, a study found that swapping the same number of calories of wheat starch with those of sugar was found to increase fasting insulin and insulin responses to a sugar load.[127] Then, in 1981, Reiser and colleagues published another study showing that when wheat starch was replaced with sugar, even when calories were kept the same, more people eventually developed diabetes/prediabetes.[128] Yet four years after this data was published, the 1985 Dietary Guidelines for Americans stated that "contrary to widespread belief, too much sugar in your diet does not cause diabetes." This was a direct contradiction to the scientific literature.

I'll be blunt: we were lied to.

The sugar industry had other strategies to keep the public naive to the harms of sugar. In the Supplemental Views to the 1977 Dietary Goals, the sugar industry stated, "It should be noted that sucrose (sugar) . . . does not displace other foods, but rather promotes their consumption. Though often referred to as empty calories, it is really *Pure Calories with No Fat and No Cholesterol*; it is an ideal energy source as an additive to other protein and nutrient providing foods [emphasis added]."

That's one Jedi-level mind trick right there.

By getting people to think of sugar as pure energy, the sugar industry helped create the general notion among the public that sugar was not inherently harmful. All we had to do was burn off the sugar calories, and we could consume as much as we wanted—and it was an appealing story to believe.

But, of course, the delusion that sugar calories are not harmful is simply not true: a sugar calorie *is* harmful, even more harmful than other carbohydrate calories, because of the way the sweet stuff affects insulin levels, brain chemistry, the immune system, inflammation, and many other physiological variables.[129] Fortunately, more and more scientists are beginning to see through the obfuscation and are becoming convinced that sugar is a factor in the development of heart disease and other types of chronic disease.[130] But back then, besides influencing the media and public perception regarding the harms of sugar, the sugar industry was undoubtedly also significantly swaying the scientific literature.

Throughout the years, the effects of conflicts of interest with the sugar industry were never quantified, until a recent systematic review of systematic reviews was published in 2013 in the journal *PLOS Medicine.* The review found that in studies with a conflict of interest with the food industry, 83.3 percent found no evidence linking sugar-sweetened beverages with weight gain/obesity. In contrast, when only studies without conflicts of interest with the food industry were analyzed, *the same percentage* (83.3 percent) found a positive association—that sugar-sweetened beverages have a definitive connection with weight gain and obesity. This one study provides just a small glimpse of how much science has likely been affected by these types of influences.[131] This was a core message I stressed during my testimony in front of the Canadian Senate regarding the harms of added sugars in our diet.[132]

The American Love Affair with Sugar

Let's take a step back and look back at the world before sugar caught us all in its thrall.

In 1776, the intake of refined sugar in the United States was just 4 pounds per person per year[133]—the equivalent of having just over 1 teaspoon of sugar in your coffee per day and nothing more—which increased to over 76 pounds of sugar by the timeframe of 1909 to 1913.[134] That's more like four frosted cupcakes per day. A similar increase in sugar intake occurred in England. In 1700, the average intake of refined sugar in England was just 4 pounds per person per year. That figure increased twenty-five-fold, to 100 pounds, by 1950.[135] During this time of skyrocketing sugar intake, the intake of salt in Europe dropped by about sevenfold, from around 70 grams per person per day in the late eighteenth century to just 10 grams in 1950.[136] The implication is clear: the intake of sugar, not salt, has paralleled the rise of chronic disease in Europe, and the same thing occurred in the United States.

In the United States, the intake of added sugars—table sugar and, later, high-fructose corn syrup—reached around 100 pounds per person per year by 1920, and stayed there until around the late 1980s, when it steadily began increasing again, to about 120 pounds in 2002. That's almost 150 grams of sugar per day, or about six of those frosted cupcakes. At that point, a staggering total of 152 pounds of total caloric sweeteners were being consumed per person per year (the 32-pound difference coming from honey, glucose, and dextrose).[137]

Thus, the intake of refined sugars in the United States increased thirtyfold from 1776 to 2002. Interestingly, this parallels the rise in chronic diseases such as hypertension, diabetes, obesity, and kidney disease.

Estimates of salt intake in the United States are harder to find, so we have to look to novel sources for clues. For example, army rations are a relatively stable reflection of the dietary intake of the times— and army rations suggest that salt intake likely declined by about 50 percent from the early 1800s to 1950.

Indeed, the army rations of the War of 1812, the Mexican War (1838), and the Civil War (1860–1861) included over 18 grams of salt per day[138]—not including the salt contained in the 20 ounces of beef, milk, beer, or rum that was also provided to these soldiers. At the close of the Civil War, the general meat ration for a soldier included $^3/_4$ pound of pork or bacon and $1^1/_4$ pounds of fresh or salt beef,[139] and the salt ration was around 18 grams per day. All of this suggests that the intake of salt during the 1800s in the United States was around 20 grams of salt per day—more than twice what we consume today.[140]

In general, the intake of salt in the United States and in Europe around 1950 and onward is probably half of what was consumed in the prior several hundred years. So it's unlikely that a rise in salt intake parallels the rise in chronic disease in the Western world. If anything, it has been inversely proportional. Since household refrigeration began in the United States (1911),[141] salt intake has been on the decline. And this would have occurred right around the time a "toxic dose" of sugar was now being consumed in the United States.

And we can trace sugar's effect on the country's health status all the way back to the 1930s. Evidence implicating sugar rather than salt as the driver of disease can be found in 1935 in the United States, a time when the percentage of deaths due to heart disease was only around 20 percent. However, by 1950, heart disease was the leading cause of death in the United States, making up around 35 percent of all deaths.[142] By 1960, that number climbed to 39 percent of all deaths (over 650,000 deaths), and arteriosclerotic heart disease made up three-quarters of these deaths. Other data show that between 1940 and 1954, death rates from coronary artery disease rose by 40 percent in men and 16 percent in women[143]—all during a time when salt intake, if anything, was *dropping*, because of the widespread use of refrigeration after 1930.

A change in the diet generally takes two to three decades to cause a rise in disease prevalence (such as heart disease)—so the "toxic threshold" of a dietary substance in the United States would have to have been reached sometime between 1905 and 1915 for there to be a dramatic rise in heart disease by 1935. In the United States, the available data does not suggest that salt hit a toxic threshold between 1905 and 1915. However, the intake of sugar did.

When we step back and look at the numbers, studying the estimates of sugar and salt consumption throughout the last several hundred years in both Europe and the United States, it becomes abundantly clear that sugar, not salt, is the likely dietary culprit contributing to chronic diseases of civilization. But just as the demonization of salt will take decades to reverse, the halo effect of unethical sugar research took (and will continue to take) years to reveal as well.

The 1980 Dietary Guidelines for Americans accepted all recommendations in the 1977 Dietary Goals—but not all targets. Sugar got the sweetest deal, as it was the only dietary factor out of the six original published goals to never receive a specific limit of intake in the Dietary Guidelines. In contrast, salt, saturated fat, and cholesterol were all given specific stringent limits for decades thereafter. Of particular note is dietary cholesterol, which, after almost forty years, has now been deemed unimportant as a cause of heart disease.[144]

In 1980, the Dietary Guidelines stated, "Estimates indicate that Americans use on the average more than 130 pounds of sugars and sweeteners a year." However, they went on to state, "Contrary to widespread opinion, too much sugar in your diet does not seem to cause diabetes" and "The most common type of diabetes is seen in obese adults, and avoiding sugar, without correcting the overweight, will not solve the problem." The 1980 Dietary Guidelines for Americans also stated that "there is also no convincing evidence that sugar causes heart attacks or blood vessel diseases."[145]

Looking back on it now, it seems as if the Dietary Guidelines were purposefully defending sugar. The overall recommendation in 1980 was to "avoid excessive sugar." By 1985, it was to "avoid too much sugar." In 1990, it was to "use sugar only in moderation," and in 1995 it was to "choose a diet moderate in sugars"—as if we *should* be eating a diet that contains moderate amounts of refined sugar. Finally, by 2000, statements such as "sugar does not cause diabetes" and "there is no proof that sugar causes diabetes" were eliminated. The advice was to "choose beverages and foods to moderate your intake of sugars."

In 2002, added sugars were finally given their first specific limit of intake since 1977. But the Dietary Guidelines did not give the limit—it came from the IOM, which published a report allowing up to 25 percent of total calories as added sugars.[146] After twenty-five years, a limit was finally placed on sugar, and yet it was more than twice the level that was allowed compared to the last recommendation decades earlier. Even by 2005, the Dietary Guidelines for Americans stated that up to 72 grams of added sugars were allowed per day (over 14 percent of total calories based on 2,000 calories per day), which adds up to 58 pounds a year.[147]

By 2010, the Dietary Guidelines for Americans technically allowed up to 19 percent of total calories (based on 3,000 calories per day) to come from added sugars (a stunning 143 grams per day). While the 2010 Dietary Guidelines did not specifically state that 19 percent of calories could be consumed as added sugars, if no solid fats are ingested, then technically this amount was allowed.[148]

Fortunately, the 2015 Dietary Guidelines Advisory Committee rights these wrongs, recommending that no more than 10 percent of calories come from added sugars (50 grams of added sugar per 2,000 calories, adding up to about 40 pounds a year).[149] The government's Nutrition Facts label will now include the specific number of grams of added sugar per serving. Perhaps the American people will finally have the information, and the guidance, they need to make the best food choices for their health. After more than two decades, the *correct* white crystal will have its bolded place of shame on the Nutrition Facts label. Unfortunately, the wrongly accused white crystal (salt) remains in bold as well. It's far past time we gave salt the justice it deserves.

Old beliefs die hard—and high-salt is still blamed mightily for contributing to heart disease in the media, in doctors' offices, and even on "heart smart" restaurant menus. Let's take a close look at the conventional wisdom behind these heart disease assertions, break them down, and settle the question—What *really* causes heart disease?—once and for all.

4

. . . .

What *Really* Causes Heart Disease?

Between their breakfasts of seaweed soup and rice and their evening meals of kalbi, barbecued beef short ribs, and a wide array of salty side dishes (banchan), the average Korean eats over 4,000 milligrams of sodium per day. They feast on tteokguk, a broth-based soup drowning in salt, or bulgogi, grilled meat marinated in a sea of sodium-packed soy sauce. They eat portions of kimchi—cabbage preserved in salt—with literally every meal.

Yet Koreans manage to somehow have one of the world's lowest rates of hypertension, coronary heart disease, and death due to cardio-vascular disease.[1] This is known as the "Korean Paradox," although you could swap out Korea for any one of thirteen other countries and get a lot more "paradoxes" regarding high salt intakes.

Three countries with the lowest rate of death due to coronary heart disease in the world (Japan, France, and South Korea) all eat a very high-salt diet.[2] The Mediterranean diet, the eating pattern now widely recommended as a heart-healthy diet, is quite high in salt (think sardines and anchovies, olives and capers, aged cheeses, soups, shellfish, and goat's milk). The French, who eat just as much salt as people in the United States, enjoy cheese, soup, traditional breads, and salted meats and have a low rate of death due to coronary heart disease.[3] Norway eats more salt than the United States yet has a lower rate of death due to coronary heart disease. Even Switzerland and

Canada have very low rates of death due to stroke despite a high-salt diet.[4]

Importantly, many of these high-salt-eating countries have very long life expectancies, including Japan, which has the longest life expectancy in the world.[5] In contrast, Latvia, with a salt intake about half that of Japan (7 grams versus 13 grams) has a death rate more than ten times Japan's.[6]

While there are undoubtedly many factors that play into these numbers—such as the fact that most of the sodium in Korea comes from kimchi (salted fermented vegetables that likely have other beneficial properties) rather than processed foods[7]—the bottom line is that even in countries known for eating a lot of salt, coronary heart disease also seems to be the *lowest* in those that consume the *highest* amounts of sodium. Among women in Korea, for example, the group consuming the highest amounts of sodium has a 13.5 percent lower prevalence of hypertension compared to the group consuming the lowest amounts of sodium.[8] And at least fourteen countries consume a diet high in salt but have a low rate of death due to coronary heart disease.[9] (See the list on page 68.) All of these countries consume the same amount of salt as people in the United States, if not more, and yet have a lower rate of death due to coronary heart disease.

We've all been told over and over again that salt raises blood pressure, which in turn increases risk of strokes and heart attacks. Looking at the population data, it's clear that high-salt diets don't seem to cause strokes and heart attacks. If anything, we see that high salt intakes lower the risk of cardiovascular disease and premature death. What's going on? How do the Koreans (and French and Japanese) get away with eating so much salt while enjoying good heart health? Why isn't all that salt raising their blood pressure? Let's take a closer look at what really happens in the body when we eat a low-salt, normal-salt, and high-salt diet.

LOW HEART DISEASE RISK IN
HIGH-SALT-CONSUMING POPULATIONS

Population: Italian nuns*

Sodium intake: ~3,300 mg sodium/day

10 fatal cardiovascular events

21 nonfatal cardiovascular events

Population: Italian laywomen

Sodium intake: ~3,300 mg sodium/day

21 fatal cardiovascular events

48 nonfatal cardiovascular events[10]

*Over 90 percent of the nuns were still alive after the thirty-year follow-up, indicating that normal salt intake does not cause hypertension and was unlikely to cause cardiovascular disease or premature death.

Population: South Korea, France, Japan, Portugal, Spain, Italy, Belgium, Denmark, Canada, Australia, Norway, Netherlands, Zimbabwe, and Switzerland[11]

Sodium intake: All consume high-sodium diets

South Korea (lowest rate of death due to coronary heart disease in the world), France (2nd lowest rate), Japan (3rd lowest rate), Portugal (6th lowest rate), Spain (10th lowest rate), and then Italy, Belgium, Denmark, Canada, Australia, Norway, Netherlands, Zimbabwe, and Switzerland[12]

All of these countries eat the same amount of salt as people in the United States, if not more, and yet have a lower rate of death due to coronary heart disease.

Japan has the longest life expectancy in the world.[13]

Latvia, with a salt intake about half that of Japan (7 grams versus 13 grams) has an over tenfold higher rate of death.[14]

Population: Korea

Sodium intake: High-sodium diet

Coronary heart disease appears to be the lowest in those who have the highest sodium intake.

In Korean women, the group consuming the highest amounts of sodium had a 13.5 percent lower prevalence of hypertension compared to the group consuming the lowest amounts of sodium. "Sodium intake has quite a limited effect on prevalence rates of hypertension or stroke."[15]

The Salt–Blood Pressure Connection

The theory, at first, made a lot of sense: excess quantities of salt cause the body to retain excess water and lead to high blood pressure in most people; consequently, reducing your salt intake will lower your blood pressure. Straight ahead, simple, logical—right?

As we've seen, it was dead wrong.

Here's the truth: normal blood pressure is less than 120/80 mmHg. But reducing your salt intake to around 2,300 milligrams per day (1 teaspoon of salt) may only lower your blood pressure by a meager 0.8/0.2 mmHg.[16] So, after enduring staggeringly bland and often debilitating salt restriction, your blood pressure may now hover around 119/80 mmHg—a mere blip, not a significant difference.

Plus, as you saw earlier, approximately 80 percent of people with normal blood pressure are not even sensitive to these meager blood-pressure-raising effects of salt; among those with prehypertension (a precursor to high blood pressure), roughly 75 percent are not sensitive to salt, and among those with full-blown hypertension, about 55 percent are immune to salt's effects on blood pressure. Indeed, even in those with hypertension (blood pressure of 140/90 mmHg or higher), reducing salt intake may only lead to a reduction in blood pressure of just 3.6/1.6 mmHg.[17]

As we've also seen, many people with normal blood pressure, prehypertension, and hypertension may even get a *rise* in their blood pressure if they restrict their salt intake.[18] This is because when salt intake is severely limited, the body begins to activate rescue systems that avidly try to retain more salt and water from the diet. These rescue operations include the renin-angiotensin aldosterone system (well known for increasing blood pressure) and the sympathetic nervous system (well known for increasing heart rate).[19] Clearly, this is the opposite of what you want to happen!

Another consequence of the low-salt diet is that your arteries can become more constricted (an increase in what's called "total peripheral resistance"), due to the depletion of blood volume.[20] To fight against this increased resistance in the smaller arteries, the heart needs to pump harder, and the pressure of the blood coming out of the heart would need to be even higher. Total peripheral resistance places additional stress on the heart and arteries, leaving you more vulnerable to chronically elevated blood pressure. In other words, low-salt diets may actually *cause* the very disease they are supposedly being used to prevent and treat, hypertension.

In short, salt's function in the body is exactly the thing it's been demonized for. "The ultimate physiological purpose of sodium intake is precisely the maintenance of blood pressure," Robert Heaney, MD, wrote in *Nutrition Today*. "Demonizing sodium is not only unsupported by evidence but is counter-physiological as well, as it ignores sodium's most basic function in mammalian bodies."[21] Sadly, because of false assumptions in the early twentieth century, the subsequent overwhelming proof of salt's innocence has been discounted. Too few people have listened to the science, too many people have argued, and too many years have been lost looking at the wrong end of the equation.

Why Did We Believe the Lie for So Long?

The public campaign against salt beginning in the late 1970s gave the impression of a consensus among scientists that salt was bad for our health. And in the public's eyes, if government and health agencies were telling people salt was bad for them, then it must be true. But unfortunately this wasn't the case. Indeed, as one editor of *JAMA* later described, "authorities pushing the 'eat-less-salt' message had made a commitment to salt education that goes way beyond the scientific facts."[22]

After Ambard and Beauchard created the great salt–blood pressure myth in 1904,[23] other early studies found increases in blood pressure—but only when giving *massive* amounts of sodium.[24] Over 18,000 milligrams of sodium (five times a normal sodium intake) had to be given in order for this effect to be seen.[25] Other publications reported similar results in normal patients: sometimes consuming up to *eight times a normal intake* did not produce hypertension in patients with normal blood pressure.[26]

Rather than admit defeat at that moment, anti-salt scientists doubled down, arguing that those studies did not last long enough to show the hypertensive effect of salt. So other authors decided to test high-salt diets for longer periods of time (several weeks rather than several days) to see if they would find increases in blood pressure. Kirkendall and colleagues studied middle-aged men with normal blood pressure and found that changing from a very-low-sodium diet (230 milligrams per day) to a high-sodium diet (9,430 milligrams per day) for four weeks led to no change in total body water or blood pressure.[27] Peripheral vascular resistance actually *decreased*, as the salt loading caused the blood vessels to relax. The authors concluded that there was no change in either systolic, diastolic, or mean blood pressure. Others had similar findings.

The bottom line was that patients with normal blood pressure had to consume an astronomical amount of salt in order to produce even mild increases in blood pressure. Additionally, high salt loads may actually cause the blood vessels to relax. Belding H. Scribner, MD, from the University of Washington School of Medicine, called our ability to handle salt amazing: "So amazing, in fact, that as much as 80 percent of a given population can handle even the highest habitual intakes of salt without danger of essential hypertension developing."[28] He called the low-salt guidelines a mistake that could "cause guilt feelings among the 70 percent to 80 percent of us who do not have to worry about salt intake." Scribner would go on to propose a more feasible solution compared to population-wide salt restriction: to identify people who were salt-sensitive and restrict sodium only in that group of the population. This at least made some logical sense.

But the idea that everyone would benefit from salt restriction was heavily promoted to the public by leading academics, government bodies, and health agencies. Even today, the notion that salt raises blood pressure in everyone is still a commonly held belief. Instead, the opposite is true: in those who have a mix of normal blood pressure, prehypertension, and mild hypertension, two-fifths (41 percent) have been found to have an *increase* in blood pressure with salt restriction.[29] And even in people with hypertension, more than one-third (37 percent) have been noted to have increases in blood pressure (of up to 25 mmHg) with salt restriction.[30] In other words, about three out of five people with normal blood pressure, two out of five people with prehypertension, and one out of three people with hypertension may have an *increase* in their blood pressure when they restrict their salt intake.

If we are truly concerned about the implications of salt intake on the health of the heart and the cardiovascular system, the elevation in heart rate with salt restriction is particularly troubling. Compared to the minuscule reductions in blood pressure, the elevation in heart rate is alarming. More importantly, those who experience a higher heart rate and blood pressure on salt restriction may have decidedly *worse* health outcomes, a fact that would affect a much larger portion of the population. Our government and health agencies have misinformed us about the supposed benefits of salt restriction; they have globalized an effect that had proven useful to only a small handful of people. (The draconian idea of "sacrificing" the majority of a population for the good of a few comes to mind!)

Yes, salt holds on to water in the body, to a certain extent—but this is actually a lifesaving property, not a harmful one. Ingesting adequate amounts of salt allows your body to maintain normal blood pressure without having to activate an arsenal of hormones to compensate. And the idea that a high salt intake causes overretention of water was also not supported by the literature.[31] In fact, studies consistently found that blood volume was not increased in patients with hypertension.[32] Even after a true blood volume expansion,[33] it takes approximately seventy-five minutes for blood pressure to increase, which is more than enough time for normal kidneys to excrete any extra salt and water to maintain normal blood pressure.

In essence, the argument that a high salt intake would lead to volume expansion (at least in people with normal functioning kidneys) didn't make physiological sense. The medical field has long known that kidneys can excrete massive amounts of salt, well beyond what we normally consume in a day. People with normal blood pressure have been found to excrete ten times a normal sodium intake, up to 86 grams of salt per day.[34] Kirkendall and colleagues found that in adults with normal blood pressure, even a *forty-one-fold* difference in the intake of sodium did not alter total body water.[35]

Perhaps the most disturbing thing about the low-salt guidelines is not how little effect they have on blood pressure when salt is restricted—but how great a *negative* effect they have on normal functioning, such as blood volume. When the intake of sodium is severely restricted, blood volume can go down by 10 to 15 percent.[36] This change indicates the body is under stress of dehydration. At that point, the body is facing an emergency, and the salt-retaining hormones are released as a last-ditch means of maintaining the body's homeostasis—to prevent a large drop in blood pressure.

In other words, a low-salt diet indicates a crisis for the body, not a recipe for optimal health. If someone were to simply consume 3,000 to 5,000 milligrams of sodium per day, those same salt-retaining hormones would stay suppressed. This fact alone is solid evidence that this level of sodium intake places the least stress on the body and is logically the body's preferred salt consumption zone to maintain homeostasis.[37]

So how did such bad science hang on for so long? The sad and simple truth is this: people were looking for easy answers. Explaining to patients and the lay public that blood pressure reductions from low-salt diets may actually indicate low blood volume and dehydration, and could place additional hormonal stress on the body, would require a great deal of detailed description. But the simple equation of Salt + Increased Thirst + Water Retention = Increased Blood Volume = Increased Blood Pressure is much easier. This simple equation just makes "logical" sense. This idea was something that the media, medical communities, the public, and government/health agencies could easily understand and get behind. And that's exactly what happened—salt was demonized as a toxic, blood-pressure-raising, addictive substance that was being consumed in massive quantities more than ever before.

Still, as convenient and simple as this explanation was, when studies proved that volume expansion could not be found in most people consuming high-salt diets, regardless of their blood pressure status, the salt–blood pressure hypothesis had to evolve in order to survive scrutiny. Rather than low-salt advocates admitting the fallacy of the core premise—"salt bad!"—they shifted their focus from blood volume to vascular resistance. Researchers began to argue that the sudden blood volume expansion that comes with higher salt intakes would lead to an increase in peripheral vascular resistance, a constriction of the blood vessels.[38]

But funnily enough, subsequent studies found that higher salt intakes *decrease* vascular resistance, causing blood vessel relaxation, while low-salt diets *increase* peripheral vascular resistance.[39] Even if someone did get a reduction in blood pressure from a low-salt diet (again, probably indicating harm from dehydration and low blood volume), there was an *increase* in peripheral vascular resistance and an *increase* in heart rate, which seemed to drastically outweigh any blood-pressure-lowering benefit.[40] Bjorn Folkow, the pioneering Swedish hypertension researcher, made a compelling case that the overall stress on the heart and arteries was from the combined effects of heart rate and blood pressure, suggesting that salt restriction increased the combined effects of heart rate and blood pressure.[41] In other words, low-salt diets would increase the overall stress on the heart and arteries and hence increase the risk of hypertension and heart failure.

Unfortunately, Folkow did not make a big splash in the media. Nor did he seem to have much influence among government or health agencies, so his ideas fell to the wayside. More importantly, a new culprit was being touted as the cause of hypertension: "natriuretic hormone."

This newly discovered natriuretic (salt-eliminating) hormone was said to help get rid of salt and water from the body by inhibiting the sodium reabsorption pump in the kidney, called Na-K-ATPase. A diet high in salt was said to lead to an increase in this hormone, causing blood vessel restriction and hypertension. Since vasoconstriction was almost always found in patients with hypertension,[42] the "natriuretic hormone" theory of hypertension gained a lot of attention. And you know what happened from here: salt took all the blame.[43]

For many years, no one really knew what exactly the "natriuretic hormone" was. However, today we know it as marinobufagenin, a steroid secreted by the adrenal glands that increases the pumping action of the heart and inhibits the sodium reabsorption pump in the kidney. However, if hypertension were caused by marinobufagenin, and salt were blamed for causing hypertension, then a diet high in salt should lead to increases in marinobufagenin. So what happens when rats are given a high-salt diet? There is indeed an increase in marinobufagenin in salt-sensitive rats, but salt-resistant rats have only "a modest increase in marinobufagenin" after eating a salty diet.[44] As we know, salt sensitivity is not a natural condition (rats needed to be bred to have this condition), so whatever defect causes salt sensitivity in humans was the problem and not salt intake per se. And the other side of the hypothesis also failed to hold up: increased marinobufagenin was supposed to lead to an increase in peripheral vascular resistance, and in humans, eating a high-salt diet does not cause this.[45] The "natriuretic hormone" theory of hypertension did not bear out in experiments.

Hiding in plain sight throughout this entire controversy? Insulin resistance and diabetes, both consistently found to coincide with both salt sensitivity and high natriuretic hormone levels. In fact, both type 1 and type 2 diabetes were associated with increased levels of marinobufagenin (the natriuretic hormone).[46] One group found that, in diabetics, disrupted Na-K-ATPase function was associated with insulin resistance, renal sodium retention, and the development of hypertension.[47] In other words, whatever was causing diabetes was also impairing the Na-K-ATPase (via increases in marinobufagenin) and causing salt-sensitive hypertension. And the dietary substance causing diabetes was . . . (drumroll, please): sugar.[48]

Before marinobufagenin was determined to be the natriuretic hormone, it was found to be significantly increased in the urine of patients with type 1 diabetes.[49]

So the inhibition of N-K-ATPase (caused by marinobufagenin) was seemingly caused by diabetes. And consuming high amounts of sugar, not salt, was consistently linked with an increased risk of diabetes.[50] Diets high in sugar were found to increase the diagnosis of diabetes or prediabetes, even when calories were held constant.[51] Thus, by increasing marinobufagenin, a diet high in sugar was the likely culprit causing hypertension as well as kidney damage and an increased risk of stroke.[52]

The idea that sugar could be causing salt-sensitive hypertension was considered nutritional blasphemy. That is, until 1988, when Ottavio Giampietro and colleagues proposed a mechanism for how diabetes causes hypertension.[53]

At the time, it was well known that people who had diabetes were also likely to have high blood pressure.[54] And Giampietro and his fellow authors knew that diabetics receiving insulin had increases in body sodium,[55] likely caused by high insulin levels in the blood, which were known to stimulate the reabsorption of sodium by the kidneys.[56] (In other words, rather than excreting the normal amount of salt in their urine, diabetics would hold on to that salt in their bodies.) Additionally, insulin-dependent diabetics were found to have high circulating levels of growth hormone,[57] which also increases sodium reabsorption.[58] Giampietro and colleagues were one of the first groups to conclude that diabetes was a state of sodium retention and decreased Na-K-ATPase activity in the heart, peripheral nerves, blood-brain barrier, and red blood cells;[59] they surmised that the sodium pump became insulin resistant in those who were diabetic, as insulin was found to stimulate its activity.[60] Thus, the idea that diabetes (or high insulin levels) was the culprit for "salt-sensitive" hypertension can be traced back as early as the late 1980s.

Interestingly, sodium in the cell was found to be higher in obese people with high blood pressure compared to those who were lean.[61] In essence, whatever causes obesity may also be increasing sodium levels in the cell.

In the 1980s, the idea that hypertension was a metabolic disorder, and in particular a state of insulin resistance, was finally beginning to gain support by many scientists.[62] Indeed, hypertension was often found to cluster in patients with high levels of glucose, insulin, and obesity.[63] And up to 80 percent of people with essential hypertension had been found to have insulin resistance.[64] Another group of authors publishing in the *New England Journal of Medicine* concluded that "essential hypertension is an insulin-resistant state."[65] Separately, John Yudkin had shown that sugar was found to increase fasting insulin levels in humans and nonhuman primates.[66] At the same time, low-salt diets were found to cause insulin-resistant blood vessels, leading to increased vasoconstriction, the same problem found in patients with hypertension.[67] Thus, it's not a huge leap to say that, even without the help of sugar, low-salt diets were probably contributing to hypertension by causing insulin resistance.

But still, old dogma dies hard, and even with this convincing new line of research, the consensus was that around 90 percent of people with high blood pressure had "essential hypertension"—high blood pressure without any known cause. These people were believed to be simply "genetically predestined" to develop hypertension—genetically susceptible to salt, not sugar.[68] Those same people were found to have increased insulin resistance, and their degree of insulin resistance was also associated with increased mean arterial pressure.[69] Having a family history of hypertension was found to more than double the risk of insulin resistance (45 percent prevalence versus 20 percent in those without a family history of hypertension). However, this created a chicken-or-egg conundrum—was it hypertension causing insulin resistance, or vice versa? In essence, those who are born to hypertensive parents have a higher degree of insulin resistance, which likely leads to higher blood pressure later in life. The authors also concluded that disturbances in these patients' ability to metabolize carbohydrates effectively could be detected well before they developed high blood pressure,[70] suggesting that insulin resistance came first, with hypertension developing later. Whatever caused the insulin resistance would then cause hypertension.

Chicken, meet egg.

These results were repeatedly confirmed in later studies:[71] children of parents with high blood pressure showed a tendency to develop insulin resistance and high levels of circulating insulin.[72]

Studies also showed that prehypertension and hypertension clustered with obesity and insulin resistance.[73] And reports began to show that salt sensitivity was common in those with obesity and hyperinsulinemia.[74] But again those old dictums held sway—obesity was considered a state of "caloric imbalance," whereas the idea that an elevated insulin level (from overconsuming sugar) could cause weight gain was not an accepted theory.

However, studies from the late 1980s up until the mid-2000s started to suggest that obesity was a state of hormonal imbalance, marked in particular by high levels of insulin, and that treating high insulin levels may treat high blood pressure. Indeed, one twelve-month study published in 2007 showed that when insulin levels were reduced as a result of lifestyle changes plus metformin (a diabetes medication), salt-sensitive blood pressure was effectively eliminated.[75] The authors suggested that the metabolic defects that appeared alongside obesity (such as insulin resistance and the activation of the sympathetic nervous system) were causing salt-sensitive hypertension, and that fixing those metabolic abnormalities corrected the salt sensitivity. Another 1989 study found that obese teenagers who lost 8 percent of their starting weight were able to correct their salt-sensitive blood pressure.[76] Animal studies extended these findings, with one showing that giving rats metformin prevented salt-induced hypertension.[77]

Another found that eating more salt *improved* the blood-pressure-lowering effects of metformin.[78]

All of this research supported the notion that insulin resistance and high insulin levels were at the center of salt-sensitive hypertension. If we treated the insulin resistance by eliminating sugar, we could fix the salt-sensitive hypertension. But still, the myth held, and lowering the intake of salt, not sugar, continued to be the focus for preventing and treating hypertension.

Even weight loss itself had been found to produce large reductions in blood pressure—even when sodium intake was not reduced.[79] One group of authors studied twenty-five obese patients in the UCLA Risk Factor Obesity Control Program who were randomized to eat a normal sodium intake of 2,760 milligrams per day or a low sodium intake of 920 milligrams per day while also losing weight. Both groups' blood pressure fell equally with weight loss. The results of the study were clear: drop the pounds, and the blood pressure would follow without having to drastically cut salt intake.

There was one final line of evidence implicating sugar as the cause of salt-sensitive hypertension, and that was cortisol. Local cortisol excess was known to lead to hypertension in those with Cushing's syndrome, chronic renal failure, and essential hypertension. And cortisol-induced hypertension was likely being confused with salt-sensitive hypertension, because as cortisol increased in the body, so did sodium, blood volume, and blood pressure. High cortisol levels were also implicated as a cause of high insulin levels, as an excess of cortisol (as seen in Cushing's syndrome) leads to abdominal obesity, glucose intolerance, hyperglycemia, hyperlipidemia, hypertension, and atherosclerosis. Undiagnosed local cortisol excess was causing hypertension—and high-salt diets continued to take the blame. It was also known that salt could raise blood pressure in animals when they were given injections of corticosteroids.[80] But if the high cortisol levels were lowered, then the hypertensive effect of salt would go away.

And so the big question: What causes high cortisol levels? And yes, you've guessed it: sugar can raise cortisol levels and hence cause salt-sensitive hypertension.[81] John Yudkin had shown this in 1974, when feeding sugar to rats increased levels of corticosterone (the equivalent to cortisol in humans) by 300 percent.[82] This was found even before insulin levels were increased, implying that elevated cortisol may actually cause insulin resistance.

Dr. George A. Perera had also written about how corticosteroids may be the underlying cause of hypertension. He showed that adrenocorticotropin hormone (ACTH), the hormone that precedes the release of cortisol and aldosterone from the adrenal gland, could increase blood pressure.[83] But it wasn't until half a century later that fructose in the brain was found to stimulate ACTH release, and thereby increase the secretion of cortisol.[84] Importantly, it was thought that fructose levels would be too low in the body for this to matter to the brain. We've since discovered, however, that fructose can be formed in the brain from glucose, particularly in states of insulin resistance.[85]

Dr. Perera also showed that low-salt diets could be dangerous in someone lacking corticosteroids. Perera wrote that reducing salt intake in a patient with Addison's disease (in which the adrenal glands produce inadequate levels of cortisol and aldosterone) led to large drops in blood pressure as well as low sodium levels in the blood and severe weakness. However, when corticosteroids were supplemented, the blood sodium returned to normal and blood pressure rebounded. Thus, it was obvious that glucocorticoids and mineralocorticoids determined the effects that dietary salt had on blood pressure and not salt intake per se.[86] And it was sugar that was found to increase glucocorticoids and hence cause people to have salt-sensitive blood pressure.

All signs have long pointed directly toward sugar—but it took us so long to see it. Part of the problem was the stubborn resistance of researchers clinging to their long-held beliefs. Another part of the problem was the willful influence of the sugar industry, deflecting attention away from the clearly guilty suspect. And the convincing

evidence disproving the salt–blood pressure theory can be seen simply by stepping back and looking at large-scale studies of whole populations. And in those studies, the findings are irrefutable.

Salt Intake and Blood Pressure: Population Studies

One of the arguments implicating salt and elevations in blood pressure was the phenomenon known as "hypertension of acculturation":
when primitive people who apparently ate little salt in their native
diet developed hypertension after acculturation, and a higher intake
of salt was thought to be the cause. Of course, these cultures also
went from eating little to no refined sugar to a diet extremely high in
refined sugar, but never mind that.

Regardless, a large body of data kept poking holes in the idea that
salt was the cause of hypertension of acculturation. For one, numerous populations that ate a high-salt diet lacked hypertension, whereas
the same could not be said for sugar. Consider the high salt intake
of these various populations and their blood pressure, shown in the
list that starts on page 82.

One of the strongest arguments supporting the notion that salt
causes hypertension and cardiovascular disease had always been from
Japan. The Japanese were known to eat lots of salt, and while in
general they had low rates of heart disease, they had a high rate of
cardiovascular conditions, such as stroke and hypertension. Indeed,
people living in Akita, Japan, were known for having a very high rate
of hypertension and death due to stroke, and they ate a lot of salt
(around 27 grams of salt per day, with a maximum intake between
50 and 61 grams) coming from miso soup, soy sauce, seasonings, and
vegetables/pickles. Salt was just one of several possible causes of their
cardiovascular disease. Researchers suggested that the high rate of
stroke in Japan (particularly in Akita) was due to other factors besides
salt, such as "an unbalanced diet consisting of polished rice and de-
ficiencies in the dietary life." Others have noted "gluttony over rice,"
"life stress such as overwork of farmers," "vitamin C deficiency in the

diet," "the quantity of silicic acid in drinking water and food," "cadmium in the intestines of widely eaten river fish of Japan," and the "sulfur/carbonate ratio of river water" as possible contributors to the high rate of death from stroke.[87] And cadmium is a likely suspect. It is estimated to contribute to 17 percent of the stroke cases in Japan.[88] Also, the low intake of saturated fat in Japan was linked to the higher rate of death due to stroke.[89]

Still, the Akita stroke rates are striking when compared with the stroke rates in Aomori, Japan, an area where the population tended to consume around 15.2 grams of salt per day. In fact, the rate of death due to stroke was more than twice as high in Akita as in Aomori. The average blood pressure in Aomori was fairly low (131.4/78.6 mmHg) and the incidence of death from stroke was only moderate,[90] with 139.2 deaths from stroke per 100,000 in those thirty to fifty-nine years old. In Akita, this number was 218.6. What was happening here?

Researchers suspected another factor at work: potassium. In a study of 1,110 adults in Aomori, Japan, an increase in apple intake was associated with lower blood pressure. Apples are a good

---

POPULATIONS THAT CONSUME AMPLE AMOUNTS OF SALT IN WHICH HYPERTENSION IS VIRTUALLY ABSENT

Population: Italian nuns
Sodium intake: ~3,300 mg sodium/day
Not a single nun with a diastolic blood pressure over 90 mmHg.[91]

Population: Italian laywomen
Sodium intake: ~3,300 mg sodium/day
Blood pressure: Progressively increased in the laywomen. The blood pressure difference was greater than 30/15 mmHg between the two groups by the end of the thirty-year study (being higher in the laywomen than the nuns).

Population: The Kuna Indians (off the coast of Panama)
Sodium intake: ~3,450 mg sodium/day (the same amount of sodium consumed in the United States today)

Blood pressure: Only 2 percent known to have hypertension. Blood pressure did not increase with age.[92]

Population: Seventh-Day Adventist vegetarians and omnivores and Mormon omnivores[93]

Sodium intake: ~3,600 mg sodium/day

Adventist vegetarians–blood pressure: 114/67 mmHg in men and 108.6/66.6 mmHg in women

Adventist omnivores–blood pressure: 121.9/72 mmHg in men and 110/66 mmHg in women

Mormon omnivores–blood pressure: 122.2/73.2 in men and 117.2/74.5 mmHg in women

Population: Java (part of Indonesia)

Sodium intake: ~3,600 mg sodium/day

Blood pressure: 124/73 mmHg in men and 128/75 mmHg in women[94]

Population: Thailand

Sodium intake: ~3,600 mg sodium/day

Blood pressure: 120/75 mmHg in men and 118/77 mmHg in women[95]

Population: Taiwan (agricultural population)

Sodium intake: ~4,000 mg sodium/day

Blood pressure: 128/83 mmHg in men[96]

Population: Samburu warriors

Sodium intake: ~4,000 to 5,000 mg sodium/day during the wet season (around five months out of the year);[97] ~3,500 to 4,000 mg sodium/day during the dry season

Blood pressure: 106/72 mmHg[98]

Population: Inhabitants of Kotyang, Nepal

Sodium intake: ~ 4,600 mg sodium/day

Blood pressure: No cases of hypertension in the men. Blood pressure did not increase with age. In the women, hypertension was extremely rare (1.4 percent). The authors concluded, "In the present study, no significant increase in systolic blood pressure with age was found in men living in Kotyang, and no hypertensive men and very few hypertensive women were detected in Kotyang in spite of taking on the average 12 g/day of salt."[99]

The intake of sugar was less than 1 gram/day in Kotyang. However, in another village in Nepal (Bhadrakali) there was a greater intake of sugar (25.5 grams/day in Bhadrakali men and 16.3 grams in Bhadrakali women). And the prevalence of hypertension was 10.9 percent in men and 4.9 percent in women.

Population: North India
Sodium intake: 5,600 mg sodium/day
Blood pressure: 133/81 mmHg[100]

Population: South India (consume less salt than North Indians yet have higher blood pressure)
Sodium intake: 3,200 mg sodium/day
Blood pressure: 141/88 mmHg[101]

Population: Apple-eating zones of Aomori, Japan (low prevalence of diastolic hypertension)
Sodium intake: ~6,000 mg sodium/day
Blood pressure: 131.4/78.6 mmHg[102]

Population: Okayuma, Japan (in the summer)
Sodium intake: ~6,000 mg sodium/day
Blood pressure: 122/75 mmHg in men and 122/72 in women[103]

Population: Bantu (rural)
Sodium intake: ~7,600 mg sodium/day
Blood pressure: 128/79 mmHg in men[104]

Population: Buddhist farmers in Thailand
Sodium intake: ~8,000 mg sodium/day
Blood pressure: No rise in blood pressure with age[105]

source of potassium. Men's systolic blood pressure tended to be over 150 mmHg when they ate no apples per day, but it dropped to less than 140 mmHg when they ate three apples per day. Researchers believed that the potassium in the apples was key here. This blood-pressure-lowering effect of apples was also confirmed in a clinical trial of thirty-eight middle-aged men and women in Akita,[106] and again in a study of Japanese patients with essential hypertension—who, despite eating approximately 15 grams of salt per day, found that their blood pressure dropped down to normal when they increased their dietary potassium intake from approximately 3 grams to 7 grams.[107] Who knew there was so much truth to the old adage about an apple a day? The problem in Akita is not the salt, but that the diet there is otherwise deficient in potassium.

This effect was also seen in Seventh-Day Adventist vegetarians, Seventh-Day Adventist omnivores, and Mormon omnivores.[108] The daily intake of sodium in these groups was between 3,500 and 3,700 milligrams, slightly higher than what the average person in the United States consumes. However, the average blood pressure in the three groups was totally normal. Importantly, the potassium intake was between 3,000 and 3,600 milligrams per day (almost twice as high as the average potassium intake in America)—providing additional evidence that potassium plays a critical role in regulation of blood pressure.

These population studies give us real-world proof that higher salt intake can be healthy—indeed, way healthier than salt restriction. But they also help us start to tease out the complexity of the factors leading to high blood pressure and stroke. Perhaps we need to shine attention on the fact that the average intake of potassium in the United States is about half that compared to what the groups studied here consumed—mostly due to lower fruit and vegetable consumption.[109] The real lesson for all of us might be that, rather than look for ways to cut salt, we could seek out ways to eat more potassium-rich plant-based foods, such as leafy greens, squash, mushrooms, and avocados. And guess what helps us to do that? Eating more salt!

How Low-Salt May Have *Created* the High Blood Pressure Epidemic

Can you begin to imagine how frustrated the researchers who openly questioned the low-salt dogma have been? They'd been proving that the low-salt emperor had no clothes for decades, but still, their voices went unheard. They knew that salt does not raise blood pressure in most of the population. They knew that even in those who have increases in blood pressure, there are benefits of a higher salt intake, such as a lower heart rate, reduced insulin levels, more balanced adrenal hormones, and better-functioning kidneys, all of which likely outweigh any risk from higher blood pressure.

At the same time, data continued to mount showing that sugar increased both blood pressure and heart rate, but it wasn't discovered until decades later that a diet high in sugar increased the risk of cardiovascular death threefold compared to a diet low in sugar. Yudkin was able to show over and over again that numerous abnormalities found in patients with coronary heart disease (elevated lipids, insulin, and uric acid and abnormal platelet function) could be caused by just a few weeks on a high-sugar diet.[110] But still, despite Yudkin's efforts, and even to this day, sugar has not been given the clear responsibility for our epidemic of cardiovascular disease. In the eyes of the public and most of the medical profession, that blame somehow— astoundingly—still lies at the feet of salt.

The Centers for Disease Control and Prevention (CDC) recently asked the Institute of Medicine (IOM) to reevaluate the evidence relating to sodium intake and cardiovascular risk, and its 2013 report found that there was no benefit for restricting sodium intake below 2,300 milligrams per day. In fact, it found that there may be adverse health outcomes.[111] Nevertheless, inexplicably, the original 2004/2005 IOM upper limit on sodium of 2,300 milligrams per day was allowed to stand and "remains the basis for federal salt policy today."[112] Even today, the leading health agencies cannot agree on what amount of salt we should be consuming—yet that *still* hasn't stopped the low-salt dogma. And the frightening conclusion to this entire controversy may end up being that a low-salt diet has contributed to, rather than helped prevent, the rising levels of heart disease in this country.

The latest double-blind, randomized studies show that low-salt diets were creating abnormalities commonly found in patients with coronary heart disease as well as the metabolic syndrome. And this effect was found in both salt-sensitive and salt-resistant patients.

Reducing salt has been found to accelerate hardening of the arteries and raise cholesterol and triglycerides in animals.[113] Salt restriction in humans with hypertension also increases plasma lipoproteins and inflammatory markers.[114] In people with chronic high blood pressure, cutting salt increased low-density lipoprotein (LDL; "bad" cholesterol) levels in the blood.[115] But other studies found that restoring higher levels of salt (going from 2 grams of salt per day to 20 grams per day for five days) significantly *lowered* plasma total cholesterol, esterified cholesterol, beta-lipoprotein, low-density lipoprotein, and uric acid in people with hypertension.[116] Even the famous DASH-Sodium trial—the foundation of the most well-known low-salt diet—found that salt restriction increased triglycerides, LDL, and the total-cholesterol-to-high-density-lipoprotein ratio (TC:HDL).[117]

Even in people who had normal weight and regular blood pressure, low-salt diets have been found to compromise kidney function, decrease high-density lipoprotein (HDL; "good" cholesterol), and reduce adiponectin, a substance released by fat cells thought to improve insulin sensitivity.[118] A Cochrane meta-analysis of almost 170 studies found that low-sodium interventions lowered blood pressure only minimally while significantly raising levels of kidney hormones, stress hormones, and unhealthy triglycerides. The authors of the Cochrane analysis (which is usually seen as the gold standard of research reviews) concluded that low-salt diets might lead to an overall negative effect on health based on increases in hormones, "bad" cholesterol, and triglycerides.[119]

Another health risk, increased blood viscosity—"thickening" of

the blood—has been thought to occur during salt restriction.[120] Increased blood viscosity, often noted in obese patients, is thought to
contribute to an increased risk of thrombotic vascular events, such as
blood clots and deep vein thrombosis.[121] Salt restriction also increases
fasting norepinephrine, a substance that increases heart rate. The
heart receives blood supply during relaxation, whereas every other
organ gets blood when the heart is contracting. So the quicker one's
heart pumps means the less time the heart is relaxed to receive blood
and, hence, oxygen. This is one reason why low-salt diets[122] have
been implicated in increasing the risk of heart attacks: by reducing
blood flow to the heart. The increase in norepinephrine on low-salt
diets may even produce cardiac hypertrophy, overgrowth of the heart,
which can lead to heart failure.[123]

Speaking for many a frustrated salt proponent, Weder and Egan
concluded in one of their papers that "the net cardiovascular risk
benefit of an average blood pressure reduction of only 1.1 mmHg
could well be more than offset by the rises in cholesterol, insulin,
norepinephrine and hematocrit resulting from salt restriction."[124] By
increasing angiotensin-II and aldosterone, low-salt diets could actually cause overgrowth of the heart and kidneys, which could lead to
heart failure and kidney disease—the very diseases we have been told
high-salt diets cause.

Weder and Egan concluded, "The potentially adverse impact of
dietary salt restriction on the risk factor profile for cardiovascular disease suggests that further studies are necessary before a reduction in
dietary salt intake can be prescribed for the general population."[125]

This was in 1991, *over twenty-five years ago.*

In 1995, Michael Alderman and coauthors openly suggested that
low-salt diets may increase the risk of cardiovascular events.[126] They
reported a more than fourfold increased risk of myocardial infarction
in men who ate the lowest amounts of salt compared to the highest-
salt-intake group.

Large-scale studies continued to emphasize these same findings.
Two large prospective European studies, which included almost four

thousand patients without prior cardiovascular disease, found a more than fivefold increase in mortality with a low sodium intake versus the highest sodium intake.[127] The Prospective Urban Rural Epidemiology (PURE) study examined over 100,000 people in seventeen countries and found that the lowest risk of death or cardiovascular events was in those consuming between 3,000 and 6,000 milligrams of sodium per day.[128] The group consuming less than 3,000 milligrams of sodium per day had the greatest risk. Graudal and colleagues performed a meta-analysis of almost 275,000 patients[129] and found that consuming between 2,645 and 4,945 milligrams of sodium per day was associated with the lowest risk of death and cardiovascular disease events. After adjusting for other confounding factors, only the group consuming less than 2,645 milligrams per day had a significant increase in all-cause mortality; this was not found in those consuming more than 4,945 milligrams of sodium per day.

Based on these data, an intake of sodium between 3 and 6 grams per day is likely the optimal range for most of us. Less than 2,300 milligrams per day or more than 6,000 milligrams per day is associated with an increased risk of death and cardiovascular events—but the risk is higher with low salt intakes than high salt intakes.

As is clear from the medical literature, as well as the population-based studies, low-salt guidelines are not "the ideal." They are not even innocuous. We may someday discover that the low-salt guidelines *created* more heart disease than they ever prevented. In the final analysis, they may even have been a contributing factor in the greatest public health challenge of our time: the rising epidemic of diabetes, caused in part by an increasingly common yet little-known phenomenon called "internal starvation."

We Are Starving Inside

There's no denying that we are in the midst of a nationwide obesity epidemic that threatens our collective health, well-being, and longevity: 69 percent of adults in the United States are now overweight or obese.[1] Obesity began to rise in the 1950s; it spiked around 1980, and the rate doubled from 1980 to 2000. Conventional wisdom blames obesity on an imbalance between our consumption of calories and our expenditure of energy—eating more calories than we burn through various activities, in other words. This is why we're often told to *eat less and move more*. As you may know from personal experience, this strategy doesn't work for everyone—or even most people.

Increasingly, alternative theories of obesity have focused on the quality of the calories we consume and how they affect us physiologically, as Gary Taubes illustrated in his book *Good Calories, Bad Calories*. Plenty of circumstantial evidence supports these contentions. For one thing, the surge in our growing girth has paralleled our increased intake of refined carbohydrates, sugar, and high-fructose corn syrup (particularly in liquid form). The sugar industry would have us believe that as long as we hit the gym to work off those calories, no harm would be done. But new research suggests that our increasingly sedentary lifestyle may actually be driven by these dietary factors, too.[2] (The potato comes before the couch.)

Given that sugar has finally been getting its due as Public Health Enemy #1, it's no surprise that sugar triggers an internal chain of events that negatively affects our waistlines and our health. But what we're just starting to realize is how a low salt intake can produce similar physiological effects. Consuming too little salt can set into motion an unfortunate cascade of changes that result in insulin resistance, an increase in sugar cravings, an out-of-control appetite, and what's been dubbed "internal starvation" (aka "hidden cellular semistarvation"), thereby promoting weight gain.[3] Someone who is overweight literally may be starving on the inside.

With internal starvation, your hormones (insulin, leptin, and others) may be working against you, essentially hijacking your appetite and revving up your desire for more unhealthy foods, and at the same time corrupting the internal processes that regulate your use of fat and protein for energy. It's as if you are no longer in charge of your eating habits and your body has gone rogue when it comes to managing its energy expenditure and intake.

When you start restricting your salt intake, your body will do anything to try to hold on to it. Unfortunately, one of the body's defense mechanisms is to increase insulin levels. It does this by creating a state of insulin resistance. When insulin resistance kicks in, the body is less able to shuttle glucose into cells, and it needs to secrete more insulin in order to control blood glucose levels. Also, remember that when a person's intake of dietary salt is on the paltry side, hormones that compensate to help the body retain salt (such as renin, angiotensin, and aldosterone) are released in greater amounts. Well, these hormones end up increasing fat absorption, too. In essence, compared to someone who hasn't slashed his or her salt intake, a low-salt diet may cause you to absorb twice as much fat for every gram you consume.[4]

This chronically elevated insulin level keeps stored fat and proteins locked away, making them unavailable to the cells that need them. When your insulin levels are elevated, the only macronutrient you can efficiently utilize for energy is carbohydrate. In effect, high insulin levels basically force you to eat more carbs because you can't readily get energy from anything else. Then, consuming high levels of refined carbs triggers greater insulin release, and the cycle repeats and reinforces itself, endlessly perpetuating the problem of high insulin levels—which, in turn, perpetuates obesity.[5]

If you slash your salt intake dramatically, you also could develop an iodine deficiency, since table salt is our best source of iodine. This is significant (and problematic!) because iodine is needed for proper thyroid function: if thyroid function dips, you could develop hypothyroidism, a condition in which your metabolic rate slows down, more fat is stored (particularly in the organs), insulin resistance develops, and weight gain occurs—yet another mechanism that can lead to internal starvation.

Plus, low-salt diets increase the risk of overall dehydration (and hence cellular dehydration), and that's a problem because generally well-hydrated cells function much more efficiently and consume less energy than dehydrated cells do.[6] The less energy that's available in your body, the greater the state of internal starvation, and the more calories you're likely to consume. Are you starting to see how low-salt diets can cause weight gain?

Even if these shifts don't lead to the accumulation of extra pounds, the result is the same: these physiological changes cause someone to become "metabolically overweight" or obese, even if it's not reflected as a higher number on the scale or as a body mass index (BMI) in the overweight or obese category. In other words, you can be "thin on the outside and fat on the inside" (what's often referred to as TOFI— aka "skinny fat"). You may be TOFI if your body weight is normal but you have a disproportionate amount of visceral fat, adipose tissue stored in your abdomen, where it is most harmful. In other words, your weight could remain within the normal range, but you could still have a dangerous buildup of fat in and around your organs as well as insulin resistance and metabolic syndrome, a cluster of conditions such as a large waistline, elevated fasting blood sugar, high blood pressure, high triglycerides, and low HDL cholesterol that raise your risk of developing heart disease, diabetes, and stroke.

With internal starvation, insulin resistance essentially degrades your body's fat metabolism system, encouraging you to overeat to compensate for all the calories that are being vectored into your fat cells and locked down there. This can make you feel like you're starving inside while you may be gaining weight at the same time. Moreover, because your body cannot access its stored energy, exercise becomes highly unappealing. Instead, your brain and body swing into calorie-conservation mode and you seek relative stillness, rather than energy-expenditure mode, because you're literally starving for usable energy. The likely result: weight gain and further body fat accumulation, another continuous cycle that perpetuates this unfortunate state of internal affairs.[7]

The concept of internal starvation was first theorized right around the time that the Salt Wars began—although it would be decades until the idea caught on. "Hypothalamic obesity," a phrase created in 1900 by French neurologist M. J. Babinski, is a condition that results from damage to the hypothalamus (the part of the brain that controls satiety and hunger), thus leading to metabolic changes, overeating, rapid, unrelenting weight gain, and insulin resistance.[8] The late Stephen Walter Ranson, MD, who was the director of the Institute of Neurology at Northwestern University, is often credited as being one of the first to suggest in the 1940s that obesity is a condition of "hidden cellular semistarvation." Ranson believed this state was triggered by a shortage of nutrients, which then forces the body to increase its food intake, reduce its energy expenditure through less physical activity, or pursue a combination of the two measures (again causing weight gain).[9] Twenty years later, Edwin Astwood, MD, an endocrinologist and physiologist at Tufts University, coined the term "internal starvation" to describe the same phenomenon.

By any name, it's a paradoxical effect that can make you wonder whether obesity leads to overeating and being sedentary, or the other way around. Increasingly, this conundrum is being addressed and studied by obesity experts and endocrinologists alike. Maybe we don't get fat because we eat too much—we eat too much because something has made us fat.

Interestingly, there's also mounting evidence that your mother's salt intake while you were in the womb can affect your risk of experiencing internal starvation once you're alive and kicking. Specifically, if your mother consumed a low-salt diet during pregnancy, you may be born into a state of internal starvation, with more fat around your organs, abnormal leptin levels, and insulin resistance.[10] A low salt intake during pregnancy may essentially program obesity in a mother's offspring from day one, according to research in animals. That's a powerful trickle-down effect, indeed!

The Salty Truth

We know that low salt intake leads to insulin resistance and increases insulin levels, and insulin resistance causes glucose to build up in the blood instead of being absorbed by the cells for energy, triggering a long, problematic chain of physiological events—excessive hunger, overeating, greater fat storage in your fat cells, and an internal energy crisis. In someone who is healthy and lean, a normal fasting insulin level is generally 5 uIU/mL or less, whereas a level just twice as high (10 uIU/mL) likely indicates insulin resistance.[11] Low-sodium diets may increase the fasting insulin level from 10 to 50 percent, which could throw someone from a healthy level to one that's trending toward diabetes.[12] One review looked at the harms of low-salt diets and reported that in studies of just one- or two-week duration, low-salt diets have an insulin-raising effect in obese patients with high blood pressure.[13] The review found that even moderate salt restriction (2 grams of salt per day) could increase insulin response to an oral glucose tolerance test in patients with high blood pressure.[14] Restricting sodium to around 460 milligrams per day (about $^1/_5$ teaspoon of salt) for one week has been found to increase fasting insulin, insulin response to an oral glucose tolerance test, fasting triacylglycerol, plasma fatty acids, and aldosterone and renin levels.[15]

We know that higher insulin levels will lead to greater fat storage, even if your overall caloric intake remains the same—and now we see that this higher fatty acid concentration in the blood may also increase damage to the arteries and blood vessels.[16] When salt restriction reduces blood circulation, less blood flows to the liver, interfering with the liver's ability to break down insulin—a possible mechanism explaining how low-salt diets raise insulin levels.

In contrast, higher-salt diets keep looking better and better. We've heard previously that eating more salt enhances the dilation of the blood vessels, especially in salt-resistant patients, an effect that sticks around for at least several months in clinical studies. Restricting your salt intake can do the opposite—constrict your blood vessels and decrease your muscles' ability to absorb glucose, which may lead to chronic high insulin and—you guessed it—increased fat storage.[17] So many pathways all lead to the same place: increased body fat.

Eighteen studies, including around four hundred patients, have looked at the effects of sodium restriction on fasting plasma insulin concentrations.[18] In one study of 147 people with normal weight and blood pressure, salt restriction caused increases in insulin, uric acid, LDL, and total cholesterol levels.[19] Fasting insulin was higher in twenty-two of the twenty-seven groups (thirteen statistically significant), unchanged in two, and lower in three (not statistically significant). Egan and colleagues found that low-salt diets increase both fasting and postglucose insulin by about 25 percent compared to high-salt diets, an effect that has been duplicated and confirmed—that is, *proven*—in many later studies and meta-analyses of randomized controlled trials.[20] Even those few people whose blood pressure might go down on low-salt diets—the "salt-sensitive" among us—experience significant increases in insulin.[21]

One of the mechanisms that could be at work here is salt's ability to actually *improve* our cells' ability to use glucose. Animal studies indicate that salt restriction worsens the body's ability to use glucose correctly while also increasing body weight, body fat, and fatty acid levels. A high salt intake likely increases the glucose transporter GLUT4 in insulin-sensitive tissues and thus allows greater glucose disposal.[22] Indeed, high-salt diets have been found to increase GLUT4 protein in both fat tissue and muscle. This is a good thing, because it allows your body to pull more glucose out of the bloodstream, reducing insulin levels and minimizing the damage that high glucose levels would have on the blood vessels. While a low-salt diet has been shown to impair insulin signaling, a high-salt diet has been proven to enhance insulin signaling.[23] Salt-restriction studies in humans have found adverse effects on glucose and lipid metabolism.[24] One animal study even found that a low-salt diet increased body weight, belly fat, and blood glucose and plasma insulin levels, while it induced insulin resistance in the liver and muscle tissue.[25]

Low-salt diets have also been found to increase liver fatty acid synthesis, which can contribute to nonalcoholic fatty liver disease (NAFLD), commonly known as "fatty liver," as well as organ fat storage, compared to a normal salt intake. Researchers found that the activity of brown adipose tissue—the "good fat" that burns calories—was reduced on a low-salt diet, indicating that low-salt diets may lower our basal metabolic rate, and possibly contribute to accelerated aging.[26]

Worse, many obese patients begin their weight-loss programs by trying to cut their carbohydrate intake. Cutting carbs causes you to become a "salt waster," excreting more salt than you would on a more balanced diet, especially when you hit ketosis (near 50 grams of carbohydrates per day or less). Thus, if you are going to cut your carbohydrate intake, you want to increase your salt intake to match the additional salt loss by the kidneys and to help prevent the subsequent rise in insulin levels to compensate for this loss. Sadly, most doctors will pair recommendations to lose weight with recommendations to reduce salt at the same time. But it appears that most people need an additional 2 grams of sodium per day compared to their normal sodium intake during the first week of carbohydrate restriction, and around an additional 1 gram of sodium per day during the second week to match increased salt losses.

THE DANGER OF DIURETICS

Thankfully, some doctors are starting to suggest increased salt as a way of short-circuiting the internal starvation cycle. Dave, an elderly retired Navy officer with a history of hypertension, diabetes, and central obesity, had recently suffered kidney failure. For years, he had been taking a diuretic medication to remove salt and water from his body in order to treat his high blood pressure. Unfortunately, the medicine caused him to experience intravascular volume depletion—a worrisome drop in the volume of blood flowing through his circulatory system—which likely worsened his kidney function. Complicating matters, Dave's intravascular volume depletion stimulated the release of salt-retaining hormones, which may have doubled the amount of fat he absorbed from his diet, increased his insulin levels, and slowed his metabolism—all the hallmarks of internal starvation.

Dave stopped taking the diuretic—but sadly, that move alone wasn't enough to fix his low-salt status or low blood volume or improve his kidney failure. So his doctor prescribed a higher-salt diet, including low-carbohydrate, salty foods like pickles and olives. After four months on the higher-salt diet, Dave's kidney function and hydration status improved and he lost 12 pounds, most of which was body fat. Increasing his salt intake combined with a reduction in the intake of refined carbohydrates improved his kidney function and internal fluid status, shifting Dave out of a state of internal starvation and into better health.

Indeed, we're finding that increasing your salt intake, even above what's generally considered a normal intake, may help improve your insulin sensitivity. One clinical trial found that compared to consumption of about 3,000 milligrams of sodium per day, those who consumed around 6,000 milligrams of sodium per day significantly lowered their glucose response to a 75-gram oral glucose tolerance test. Moreover, the researchers found that when diabetic patients were placed on the higher-sodium diet, their insulin response improved. The authors were quite emphatic and suggested that some people even supplement with sodium, stating that "an abundant sodium intake may improve glucose tolerance and insulin resistance, especially in diabetic, salt-sensitive, or medicated essential hypertensive subjects."[27]

We know that low-salt diets seem to cause your fat cells to become resistant to the effects of insulin,[28] which in turn increases the level of glucose in the blood and causes oxidative stress, inflammation, and damage to your arteries, as well as further insulin resistance. It's a vicious cycle of internal starvation. Doctors have known for decades that giving people diuretics, which help the body get rid of salt, can also promote insulin resistance and diabetes. Well, when you restrict your salt intake, you are essentially deriving the same detrimental physiological effects as if you were placed on a diuretic medication.[29]

So, to recap this madness:

- Insulin resistance and higher insulin levels are likely physiological adaptations to salt restriction.
- Insulin helps the kidneys to reabsorb salt, a compensatory mechanism to help the body retain more salt.
- The elevation in insulin levels makes us fatter and shifts us further into internal starvation.
- Our skeletal muscle and fat cells become insulin resistant to prevent the higher insulin levels from causing our blood glucose level to drop too low (hypoglycemia), which could be potentially fatal.

- This leads to higher glucose and fatty acid levels circulating in the body, which damages blood vessels and causes more fat to be stored in and around our vital organs instead of being stored where fat should be—in our fat cells.
- Eating too little salt, rather than too much, triggers this entire unnecessary, self-reinforcing, ever-downward health spiral.

At any moment, you can begin to reverse this downward spiral—with more salt! Getting enough salt can also help you get a grip on your sugar cravings and maintain an appropriate fluid balance in your body, which will help with proper metabolic function.

The Sugar Connection

As important as it is to increase salt to prevent internal starvation, it's even more important to avoid sugar. We all know that calories from sugar are especially detrimental when it comes to our ability to manage our weight and overall health. This is partly because a greater intake of sugar calories stimulates more insulin resistance and more fat storage than other types of calories do, even when the total calorie intake remains the same.[30]

Excessive consumption of fructose can cause too much fat to accumulate in the liver, which causes this vital organ to become resistant to insulin, thereby setting you up for overall insulin resistance throughout your body.[31] A high fructose intake can also decrease the adipose tissue's fat-storing capacity, slamming that fat into and around organs like your heart, pancreas, and liver. (Indeed, by overconsuming fructose you hit the liver with fat storage from two different directions.) This is harmful to your health on so many levels because it causes chronic inflammation and oxidative stress, among other detrimental effects.[32] What's more, letting your sweet tooth get the upper hand on your diet can also damage mitochondria, the power source in your cells, which leads to a decrease in ATP that in turn increases your hunger and leaves you with no energy for exercise.[33] Those high glucose levels in the blood even pull water out of the cells, causing cellular dehydration. The water that was essentially stolen from your cells and pushed out into your blood—a phenomenon that has traditionally been blamed on salt, by the way—leads to a lower salt level in your blood.

In essence, a high-sugar diet increases your need for salt by diluting its level in your blood.[34] And yet this is one more way to illustrate how more salt can help us: eating enough salt to satisfy our salt cravings may just be the key to kicking our sugar cravings for good.

6

· · · · · · · · · · · ·

Crystal Rehab: Using Salt Cravings to Kick Sugar Addiction

Salt is one of our five innate taste sensations, and with good reason: besides making food taste good, we've seen how vital salt is to our health. Fortunately, the human body has a built-in system—a "salt thermostat"—that helps us get just the right amount. Our salt thermostat signals the brain to seek more salt when we need more to meet our physiological needs, as well as to stop when we have enough to fulfill our biological functions. This built-in system helps regulate our internal fluid-salt-electrolyte balance and resets it when necessary— and it's all taken care of automatically, without any effort on our part.

Sugar is another matter entirely. Unlike cravings for salt, which are controlled by our bodies' innate need, sugar cravings are produced by either psychological desire (and, in some people, addiction) or physiological cravings (in response to low blood sugar from prior sugar overload). They're not signs that your body actually *needs* sugar—your body actually requires zero dietary sugar to survive. In scientific terms, the intake of salt is a negative feedback system (at a certain point the body tells itself to reduce intake), whereas sugar is a positive feedback system (the more sugar you eat, the more you want, crave, and therefore keep eating). While one is the sign of a biological mandate, the other can become a self-inflicted, life-shortening, extremely damaging addiction.

Luckily for us, relearning how to listen to one has the power to help heal us from the other. It's time to set the record straight about the health-protecting, lifesaving nature of salt cravings—and drop the guilt for good.

Is Salt Addictive?

Salt tastes good—and eating it makes our bodies feel good. When we need more salt, we crave more salt. During low salt intake, you are more sensitive to the taste of salt—salt will literally taste saltier. Here's why: the flavor of salt is a signal to your body, and if you weren't able to detect salt during periods of low intake, you could possibly die. When you reduce the amount of salt you consume, your ability to detect salt is *enhanced*, an evolutionary adaptation that has ensured the survival of numerous species for millions of years. When foods taste saltier to you, that's your body sending you a direct message: "Hey, check this stuff out! You need more of this!" But you honestly don't need to be concerned about overeating salt. If you habitually add salt to your food, the worst that could happen is that your taste buds get used to that level of saltiness—but even if you happen to binge on salt, we know that our kidneys simply reabsorb less. No harm, no foul. In fact, as we've seen, eating higher levels of salt may even be healthier in the long run.

More often than not, salt cravings suggest that your internal fluid-salt-electrolyte balance is out of whack. Caffeine increases sodium excretion, which could cause java junkies to develop an increased penchant (and a physiological need) for salt. The same is true of athletes and avid exercisers: if someone exercises for an hour, they may lose around 2 grams of sodium, so their intake would need to be higher in order to replace what was lost.

This is all established science—so why is the "salt addiction" myth still with us? The origin of the myth all goes back to the moment we stopped looking at salt as an essential, life-giving force—and started seeing it as a hedonistic indulgence, a human appetite to be managed as opposed to trusted.

When Salt Became a Spice

M. Lapicque, who studied the salt habits of native Africans of the Angoni district,[1] was first credited in 1896 with proposing the idea that salt was a condiment, similar to pepper, curry powder, paprika (capsicum), and other flavoring agents, its main purpose being a "gustatory stimulus."[2] This idea stems from the fact that when salt is introduced to low-salt-eating natives, their salt intake increases. Anti-salt evangelist Graham MacGregor was one of the biggest promoters of the idea that "the 'need' for salt is a habit [a mild form of addiction] that can be changed by gradual reduction in the salt content of the food consumed."[3] And other low-salt advocates similarly believed—and still do believe—that salt is mildly addictive. For example, fathers of the 1977 low-salt recommendations, George Meneely and Harold Battarbee, were highly influential in promoting the idea that salt is addictive. These authors believed that the intake of salt was "induced" from its "noxious effects beginning in childhood, when habits of excess salt consumption are acquired at the family table, and are perpetuated by continuing habit."[4]

This idea actually stemmed from our old pal Lewis Dahl, who, like Meneely and Battarbee, viewed salt as "a condiment, not a requirement."[5] Lewis Dahl suggested that salt intake was induced because of its ubiquity in the food supply. He suggested that if salt was provided in lower amounts, we would adapt and consume less, and if given more salt, we would rapidly become accustomed to it and begin eating a diet higher in salt. Meneely and Battarbee followed Dahl's lead and suggested that "salt appetite is induced rather than innate and that like salt intake, appetite for salt bears no necessary relation to requirement." So, in essence, the idea that salt is addictive can be traced back to those few low-salt advocates who brought us the low-salt guidelines to begin with—another commonly held belief that comes from their "expert opinion" rather than sound science.

Our "hunger" for salt bears the most physiological resemblance to our thirst for water—how much we take in is controlled by how much we need. In summer, we drink more water because we lose more in our sweat; in winter, our water intake goes down.[6] We adjust water intake by listening to our thirst. Salt consumption works exactly the same way. Indeed, numerous experiments have found that animals who are deficient in salt will increase their intake once it's available—which is why animals are drawn to a salt lick.[7] The same happens in humans who have been depleted of salt (such as athletes on a hot day or someone receiving dialysis).[8]

In essence, your body knows better than the experts how much salt it needs—and telling someone to restrict their salt intake is akin to telling someone to restrict their water intake when they are thirsty. It just makes no biological sense.

So how did this myth get started? Some experts used population data to suggest that salt intake will increase when it is introduced to societies that do not use a lot of salt. Norman K. Hollenberg of Harvard Medical School termed it a "habituation" that can develop with salt intake, similar to what happens with alcohol, tobacco, and coffee, all of which are habit-forming. However, this increased intake does not mean salt is habit-forming—it's actually evidence that if enough salt is available, people will consume more, but only up to a physiologically determined set point, one that provides ideal health and longevity. Indeed, when salt is freely accessible, people across numerous populations tend to eat an amount that stays within a remarkably narrow range, generally between 3 and 4 grams of sodium per day.[9] When salt is freely available, even animals consume an amount almost exactly proportional to humans' instinctive intake.[10] This consistency supports the idea of an evolutionary "salt set point" that resides in both humans and animals. Our salt intake is unconsciously controlled by our internal salt thermostat.

What may look from the outside like salt "addiction" may actually be a reflection of the flux in salt storage. Interestingly, salt can be stored in the skin—similar to the way a camel stores fat in its hump, but distributed widely and invisibly—via a mechanism that appears to be controlled by certain hormones that are produced within the body. Some have proposed that aldosterone increases those salt stores in the skin, whereas cortisol may deplete those stores.[11] (Recall that aldosterone also helps the body retain salt during salt depletion.) When we aren't eating enough salt, aldosterone increases, which in turn stores salt in the skin. People who have consumed low-salt diets their entire lives, such as those in primitive societies, automatically switch over to eating more salt once it's introduced, and the higher salt intake may cause the body to lose some of its salt stores in the skin. The reduced amount of salt in the skin may be a signal to continue to eat the salt in the range of 8 to 10 grams per day. In essence, the fact that certain low-salt-eating people begin to consume more salt once it's introduced may have nothing to do with salt being addictive—and everything to do with human physiology. They're simply eating more because those hidden salt stores in the body have gone down because of the increased salt supply in their environment.

Also, don't forget that compared to a low-salt diet, a normal-salt diet seems to place less stress on the body—so instead of the body continuously trying to retain more salt through the chronic activation of salt-retaining hormones (which requires a lot of energy), it can simply get the salt it needs through the diet and not worry about having to reabsorb as much at the kidneys. And let's face it, why would the body choose to take in less salt if doing so puts more stress on its organs? Indeed, our internal salt thermostat seems to drive us to consume an amount of salt that places the least stress on our body.

Certain individuals have "less desire" for salt after reducing their intake, a phenomenon that has been proposed as proof that low-salt diets are ideal.[12] But this theory has never been proven to be true; even if some people eat less salt upon its restriction, this is undoubtedly a conscious choice. In fact, even if there is a reduction in the desire for salt with salt restriction, this is due to the kidneys shutting off salt excretion (the kidneys try to hold on to every filtered milligram of sodium on low-salt diets). Furthermore, only a small percentage (around 25 percent) of the population can even drive their salt intake down to what most guidelines recommend.[13] The body seems to "fight" salt restriction with all its might because of the additional stress placed on it by salt restriction. Those who seem to be consuming extremely high amounts of salt (putting salt on every meal they eat) may unconsciously be protecting their optimum blood volume.[14] So the next time you find yourself looking at someone with those "judgy eyes" across the dinner table or at a restaurant as they sprinkle loads of salt on their food, you should instead think to yourself, "That person's body is telling them they need more salt."

So if your body were to become depleted in salt, how would it know? And more importantly, how would it force you to behave to replace what was lost?

The Dark Side of Low-Salt Eating

The body has a very elegant way of ensuring that you replace any lost salt: by making your brain's reward system hypersensitive and allowing it to receive more pleasure from eating salt. This "sensitization" occurs during salt depletion, giving you a greater craving for salt so you seek it out, and then helping you experience increased reward when you eat a lot of it.[15] Salt depletion simply makes us like salt better.[16] This survival mechanism developed over 100 million years of evolution and has ensured the survival of almost every single species since then.[17] If our body could not enhance the brain's craving and reward for salt during states of deficit, our species (as well as others) would have become extinct long ago.

However, there is a downside to this enhanced reward in the brain when we restrict our salt intake: the same sensitization that drives you to seek out and consume more salt could also prime your brain for other addictions. By turning up the volume on your reward circuitry, your brain may experience greater pleasure when consuming other dietary substances that trigger the brain's reward system. This priming could create problems with addictive substances, especially refined sugar and drugs of abuse, increasing their addictive potential.[18]

It's not too much salt that creates "salt addiction." It's salt restriction, which increases our risk of salt depletion, that can produce changes in the reward center of the brain. Restricting salt leads to structural modifications in the nucleus accumbens that cause the brain to get a greater reward or "high" from salt. These modifications resemble the changes that occur in people who have become addicted to drugs of abuse, and this sensitization can be hijacked by other substances of abuse.[19]

Sounds amazing, doesn't it? That an enhanced "hunger for salt," born during times of salt depletion, may "cross over" and enhance our reward from refined sugar and drugs of abuse? But the evidence in the literature strongly supports this notion. For example, sodium depletion has been found to cross-sensitize with amphetamine, a drug also known to cross-sensitize with cocaine.[20] Cross-sensitization is a phenomenon that generally only occurs between drugs of abuse, in which the use of one drug leads to enhanced effects (and increased abuse potential) of the other.[21] In this case, *sodium depletion itself* is acting like a substance of abuse, increasing the reward and abuse potential of other substances of abuse. Indeed, this shared brain pathway was shown in a 2009 study from the University of Florida College of Medicine in Gainesville. Investigators were looking into the Salted Food Addiction Hypothesis, which proposes that salty food acts in the brain like an opioid drug, stimulating our brain's receptors and producing pleasurable reward sensations and cravings when salty food isn't available.[22] The researchers found that salty food has a slight appetite-stimulating effect in people who are dependent on opiates, but not in nonaddicts. This point underscores the shared pathways in the brain and really highlights how dangerous salt restriction can be: by making the brain's addictive pathways more sensitive, salt restriction likely also makes people more susceptible to dangerous addictive drugs and food addiction.

Restriction-induced periods of enhanced salt cravings do not seem to lead to prolonged overconsumption—they seem to last only until

the salt depletion has been corrected. And once it is corrected, in-
hibitory signals will turn off the "liking" for salt and turn on an "aversion" signal.[23] It has been postulated that a high salt intake during
times of repletion causes the "salt receptors on the tongue to 'flip'

REVERSING INTERNAL STARVATION

Consider Julie, an elderly retired social worker with a rich
family life (including grandkids), who goes to the gym five
days a week. Because she does indoor cycling three or four
times a week, her legs are slim and strong and her weight is
in the normal range—so she couldn't understand why she'd
gained a fair amount of fat around her midsection recently.
Two years ago, she went to the doctor for a checkup and
learned that the statin drug she'd been taking to control
her slightly high cholesterol could increase her risk of developing diabetes; worse, the results of her lab work revealed
that her fasting blood sugar level was already in the prediabetes zone (elevated but not high enough to be considered
full-blown diabetes).

Julie's story has a chicken-or-egg element because it
isn't clear whether it was the statin or her diet that raised
her blood sugar, but the result was the same: she was in a
state of internal starvation and at increased risk of developing type 2 diabetes. At her request, her doctor agreed to
take her off the statin on the condition that she modify her
diet further—opting for low-glycemic (lower-carb) foods—
and begin doing strength training three times a week in addition to her aerobic workouts. Since then, she has slimmed
down, especially in the abdomen; she has gained energy;
and her fasting blood sugar has improved—signs that she
is no longer in a state of internal starvation.

---

from positive to negative . . . quite unlike the response of the other four basic taste sensors and thereby tends to decrease intake of salty foods."[24] (Behold the salt thermostat at work!)

We live in a society where substances of abuse are readily accessible. Almost thirty thousand people in the United States die every year from overdosing on prescription opioids, cocaine, and heroin.[25] Given the very real death toll of this staggering epidemic, if salt depletions and low salt intakes increase the potential to abuse addictive substances, we need to seriously ask ourselves: Do the hypothetical and largely disproven "benefits" of restricting our salt intake really outweigh the proven, multiple, life-threatening risks? Or is it time to hold our public health officials accountable for their willful disregard of decades of scientific evidence, and protect future generations from these needless risks?

Following the low-salt advice could be "priming" or "sensitizing" our brains for an excessive reward from refined sugar and drugs of abuse. In essence, our evolutionary hardwired defense mechanism to survive times of salt depletion may now be working against us, increasing our risk of becoming hooked to addictive substances. And the longer we try to adhere to the low-salt advice, the more intensively we may be increasing our risk of abusing refined sugar and drugs of abuse. We need to do everything we can to protect our innate salt thermostat from getting derailed.

From Cradle to Grave: How Our Salt Thermostat Gets Derailed

Two of the most common ways our natural salt thermostat can get hijacked are, first, to become salt-depleted early in life; and, second— you guessed it—to follow the low-salt guidelines. And it all starts at the very beginning, in the womb.

Let's say your mother consumed too little salt during pregnancy, thinking she was doing the right thing for herself and her baby. As

a fetus, your body would develop in a salt-deprived state, and the dopamine receptors in the reward center of your brain would become
highly sensitized to salt, causing you to get amplified gratification
from eating salt. Studies have noted that a low salt intake in pregnant
mothers may cause offspring to eat and crave more salt throughout
childhood and adulthood.[26] The increase in salt appetite seems to
help ensure the survival of offspring during further sudden dehydration events (such as dramatic sweat loss on a hot day). Unfortunately,
it may also predispose you to addiction to substances of abuse.

This adaptation started out well. Fessler introduced the idea that
there is a prenatal "early calibration system" for salt preference. He
believed that "complex neurophysiological machinery" was responsible for creating our innate set points for salt intake, and they helped
us maintain homeostasis later in life. These set points might have
helped save our ancestors from dangerous bouts of dehydration from
diarrhea and vomiting due to intestinal infections. Then, natural
selection would ensure that this adaptation would be passed on to
future generations.[27]

As evolution continued, however, this adaptation would eventually make us a bit more vulnerable in modern life. Because salt depletion early in life (in utero or shortly after birth) seems to predispose
offspring to become drawn to eating higher levels of salt, they will
probably also have an increased risk of becoming addicted to drugs of
abuse as well as refined sugar due to chronic activation of the brain's
reward system.[28]

Unfortunately, many well-intentioned pregnant and nursing
mothers follow the low-salt advice given to them by their doctors—
and, as a consequence, they may be predisposing their children to
salt, sugar, and drug addiction. This is just another example of how
low-salt advice may lead to the exact outcomes that it is being touted
to prevent. Talk about unintended consequences!

When it comes to the intake of salt, your body knows best. Eating
the level of salt that your body drives you to consume, rather than
trying to consciously restrict your salt intake, will help ensure that

you avoid harms during salt depletions, and by doing so may help you prevent problems with sugar and other drugs of abuse.

Salt and Anxiety

A 2011 study from the University of Haifa in Israel suggests that a high salt intake may help buffer the effects of stress, serving as an *adaptive* coping mechanism for dealing with psychological and emotional adversity. As part of the same line of study, the researchers also found that decreased consumption of sodium-rich foods caused anxiety in subjects when they were presented with mental challenges.[29] Similarly, researchers at the University of Iowa found that when rats are deficient in sodium chloride (table salt), they shy away from normally enjoyable activities, suggesting that salt has a positive effect on mood.[30] Low-salt diets can cause tremendous sacrifice and general misery for those who attempt to follow them. Pines and colleagues have even suggested that low-salt diets may induce serious anxiety, hypochondriasis, and invalidism.[31] In other words, people feel anxious and ill on low-salt diets.

Some people may turn to sugar to help them cope. The increased psychological anxiety from consuming diets low in salt may lead to sugar cravings, as sugar triggers neurochemical release in the brain that may help people temporarily "manage" their anxiety.[32] It's commonly believed that consuming sugar has a positive effect on mood, but it's a fleeting lift at best. If people opt to reach for sugar rather than salt, they may find themselves becoming dependent on sugar as a short-term stress fix. The negative effect of that coping mechanism would only be heightened on a low-salt diet, leading to a perpetual cycle of "medicating with sugar"—and, eventually, sugar addiction.

How Low-Salt Eating Makes Sugar More Addictive

When left to their own devices, we've seen how animals (including humans) consume just the right amount of salt, and then stop. Either the salt craving goes away or our bodies excrete any excess. Nothing remotely similar occurs with sugar. While some people normally eat just a little bit of sugar, a large and growing group of people, particularly kids, consume refined sugar and/or high-fructose corn syrup in massive amounts, without an "off" switch. In fact, John Yudkin, MD, the founder of the Department of Nutrition in Queen's College of London and an early anti-sugar activist, noted that up to 52 percent of total calories come from sugar in adolescents age fourteen to eighteen.[33]

And unlike cravings for salt, which are controlled by our bodies' innate need for it, sugar cravings are produced by either a psychological desire or a physiological dependence on it. Regardless of how powerful these cravings are, they're not signs that your body actually needs sugar! As we saw in the last chapter, consuming lots of sugar can contribute to the state of internal starvation, stimulating your appetite and nudging you to eat more—and more sweets, in particular. One of the worst offenders in triggering internal starvation is fructose, which is mainly derived from sugar beet, sugarcane, or corn. When fructose is stripped out of these naturally high-carbohydrate foods, then boiled down to concentrated form and added to other foods, it becomes more addictive and harmful than in its original state. If it seems crazy to think of a plant product becoming an addictive drug, think of cocaine from coca leaves or heroin from poppy seeds/pods—in essence, these are all concentrated addictive substances from plants.[34]

With salt, we don't see a continuous escalation in its intake. Contrast that with sugar. After the introduction of sugar in the diet of both animals and humans, scientists have charted a definitive thirty-fold escalation in its intake, with evidence of bingeing, tolerance, and structural changes in the brain in response to that consumption—all key criteria of addiction.[35] Consider alcohol: some people will become alcoholics and will consume massive amounts, while others will not. English poet John Gower invented the term "sweet tooth" in his criticism of the indulgences of courtly life, and he understood back in the late 1300s that it was not normal to indulge in sugar or sweetness.[36] Indeed, once a "sweet tooth" develops, people favor foods that once tasted too sweet, and what used to taste rather pleasant may now seem bland, and perhaps even slightly bitter. When the taste receptors change because of consuming a diet high in added sugars, a person may find it more difficult to enjoy nonsweet foods, precipitating a further sweetening of the diet.

Once upon a time, our taste for sweet foods was functional because it ensured that our ancestors would consume enough calories and nutrients from naturally sweet foods like berries and other fruits. But in our modern food supply, the natural sugar from whole foods has been extracted and stripped of its inherent fiber, water, and phytonutrients until all that's left is a refined white crystal or chemically produced syrup. Unfortunately, this sweetening does not generally result in an increased consumption of fruits or sweeter vegetables—but rather an increased consumption of refined sugars. When we consume packaged foods and beverages that are loaded with this processed sugar, our bodies absorb it rapidly and our brain registers an off-the-charts reward, thanks to an intense release of natural opioids and dopamine that can override our self-control mechanisms. Indeed, brain scan research conducted on humans and animals has shown that processed foods containing large amounts of refined sugar stimulate the brain's reward centers, causing them to light up on PET scans like pinball machines, just as addictive drugs like heroin, opium, and morphine do.

People can also develop a tolerance to sugar so that they need more and more of it to satisfy their sweet tooth. And those who are hooked on sugar can experience mood changes and bingeing behavior—as well as withdrawal symptoms when they're suddenly cut off from or go too long without consuming sugar. As they withdraw from sugar, people may even have ADHD-like symptoms (from a depletion of dopamine in the brain), such as being unable to concentrate or think straight, or experience shakiness, jitteriness, sweating (from low blood sugar, a result of physiological withdrawal and dependence), and anxiety.

Do any of these symptoms sound familiar?

In fact, people with obesity, ADHD, and drug addiction to cocaine and heroin share a similar brain signature. All three have the same downregulation of the dopamine D2 receptors in the brain, indicating a lack of normal dopamine function in all three conditions. As dopamine is the "reward neurotransmitter," people who have a sugar dependence may experience a mild depression when they eat less sugar, which needs to be subsequently "treated" by consuming more of the sweet stuff. The intense release of dopamine that follows a person's first dose of sugar causes a short burst of "happiness," followed by a period of "depression," which can then be "treated" with sugar . . . and the cycle is often repeated throughout the course of the day.

While this emotional dependence can be a hard habit to break, the body can develop a state of physical dependence. People with insulin resistance release an excessive amount of insulin when they eat sugar, causing large drops in blood sugar levels, which can lead to shakiness, jitteriness, sweating, palpitations, and anxiety—nudging them back toward the sugar to "cure" their ills. If indulged regularly, this could create a vicious cycle of continued sugar intake (and true sugar dependence) in order to treat the low blood sugar levels. As many as 110 million Americans have some form of insulin resistance,[37] so much of the population is not only at risk for type 2 diabetes but is likely also at risk for sugar addiction.

Addiction to sugar may even be more intense than addiction to other drugs of abuse. Studies have found that when rats are addicted to cocaine, if they're given a choice between cocaine and sugar, they will opt for the sugar instead, likely because the reward from sugar surpasses that of even cocaine.[38] Some of the best proof we have of sugar's true addictive power is how that addiction can be treated. Drugs that are designed to block the brain's opiate receptors and are used to treat opiate addiction (in those hooked on heroin and morphine) may also help with dependence on sugar. (See the table that follows for the shared features between addictive drugs and sugar, and the list following that for a possible effective strategy that the U.S. Food and Drug Administration [FDA] should consider approving for the treatment of sugar addiction.) People don't get strung out on sugar like they can on illicit drugs—sugar doesn't distort your perception of reality and although they may feel like it, nobody is *literally* going to kill for a cookie—but they can certainly experience pronounced withdrawal effects.[39]

Shared Features between Addictive Drugs and Sugar [40]

Neurochemical/Behavioral Effects	Addictive Drugs	Sugar
Withdrawal upon removal	+++	+
Withdrawal from an opiate-antagonist	+++	++
Reward upon consumption (persistent and intense release of opioids and dopamine after administration, leading to behavioral reinforcement)	++	+++
Increase in dopamine D1 receptor binding	NCD	NCD
Decrease in D2 receptor binding	NCD	NCD
Decrease in D2 receptor mRNA in the nucleus accumbens	NCD	NCD
Increase in μ-opioid receptor binding	NCD	NCD
Dopamine/acetylcholine imbalance upon naloxone withdrawal	NCD	NCD
Dependence on endogenously released opioids	+++	++
Sensitization to stimuli acting upon D1 and μ-opioid receptors (likely leads to addiction)	++	++
Dependence due to a low dopamine state in the brain	+++	++

+ moderate, ++ strong, +++ very strong, NCD–no comparative data

Note: These ratings do not necessarily indicate the exact strength of effect; rather, they are meant as a general comparison.

**A POSSIBLE TREATMENT STRATEGY FOR
SEVERE SUGAR ADDICTION**

As a doctor of pharmacy, I have a unique perspective on the power of pharma-
ceuticals to help with our most entrenched health problems. The medications
buprenorphine and naloxone are labeled only for the treatment of opiate dependence, but I believe the FDA should consider this prescription treatment strategy
for treating severe sugar addiction. (Note: These medications are considered controlled substances, so only certified prescribers can write prescriptions for these
medications.)

Induction treatment of sugar addiction
• At first sign of sugar withdrawal, give buprenorphine (a partial opioid
antagonist/agonist), sublingual tablet, 8 mg on day 1, 16 mg on day 2

Maintenance treatment of sugar addiction (generally day 3)
• Start with Suboxone (buprenorphine plus naloxone), 2 mg/0.5 mg sublingual
films or tablet (1 film or tablet under the tongue once to twice daily)

• Suboxone may induce withdrawal if you try to ingest sugar (you may not get the
sugar high, which may help maintain a sugar-free diet); a target of 16 mg/4 mg for
maintenance is suggested; titrate in 2–4 mg buprenorphine increments

As we talked about previously, excess consumption of refined sugar,
particularly of fructose-derived sweeteners such as sucrose and high-
fructose corn syrup, can also trigger resistance to the satiety hormone
leptin, throwing your appetite and your body's fat-regulation system
out of whack.[41] Normally, leptin, which is released by our fat cells,
crosses the blood-brain barrier and binds to receptors in the appetite-
regulating center of the brain, helping regulate your calorie intake
over the long haul. Leptin tells you to stop eating and to increase your
physical activity when appropriate; it also activates the central nervous system, stimulating fatty tissue to burn fat for energy. So there's a
harmful double whammy that occurs when someone becomes leptin
resistant. The brain believes the body is starving, triggering continued hunger and calorie intake—most often in the form of those fast-
acting carbs because, remember, these are the only macronutrients
your cells can burn efficiently while insulin levels are raised and your

body is in "internal starvation."[42] A consistently high sugar intake will diminish your appetite for nourishing foods, and the changes that occur in the brain during this overconsumption of refined sugar can lead to sugar dependence, sparking intense cravings and binge-ing, and then withdrawal symptoms when you don't consume sugar on a regular basis.[43] And all of these mechanisms become even more pronounced in the absence of sufficient salt.

For these and many other reasons, it's clear that sugar, not salt, can be addictive. Sadly, the staggering availability and consumption of sugar makes us sitting ducks for sugar addiction—while the bias against salt could be blocking a cure we so desperately need. It's time for us to get savvy about salt: who (really) needs less, who really needs more, and how we can look to salt's wildly undervalued powers to help us recapture our nation's lost health.

How Much Salt Do You Really Need?

As with many things in life, there's an optimal range of salt consumption. That ideal varies somewhat from one person to another. Advocates of salt restriction don't consider how much sodium we need to *thrive*; they focus only on our minimum requirement in order to survive. So how do you make sure you get enough—but not too much?

The good news is that many healthy people needn't worry about hitting salt overload. The body takes care of any excess. Scientific research suggests that the optimal range for sodium intake is 3 to 6 grams per day (about $1^1/_3$ to $2^2/_3$ teaspoons of salt) for healthy adults, not the 2,300 milligrams of sodium (less than 1 teaspoon of salt) per day that's commonly advised. And some people need even more.

But before we dive into figuring out your unique ideal salt intake, I should clarify that a few of us should be concerned about consuming and retaining too much salt, such as people who have the following conditions:

- Hyperaldosteronism (an aldosterone disorder that involves increased secretion of the salt-retaining hormone called aldosterone)
- Cushing's disease (a disorder of the pituitary gland that causes high cortisol levels in the blood)

- Liddle syndrome (an inherited form of high blood pressure that causes excess reabsorption of sodium in the kidneys)

These folks should monitor and possibly limit their salt intake because they may be especially sensitive to the negative effects of sodium on their blood pressure. But even for these individuals, salt isn't the main issue; if you treat the underlying disease effectively, you can treat the excessive salt retention.

Most of us, by contrast, have a number of strong defense mechanisms that kick in if we start to retain excess salt in the body. If our blood and fluid levels of sodium get high, we start reabsorbing less salt from the kidneys and absorb less salt from the foods we eat—our intestines make some of the adjustment for us. If sodium begins to accumulate, our bodies also tend to harmlessly shunt excess sodium to the skin or organs. Recent research from the Interdisciplinary Center for Clinical Research at the Friedrich-Alexander-University Erlangen-Nuremberg in Germany has shown that our bodies have significant sodium stores in our skin, which seem to help prevent dehydration and to block infectious organisms from entering the skin.

Indeed, we may find that our bodies need more salt (even more than 3 to 6 grams of sodium per day) than ever before because of our modern health and lifestyle habits, such as the following:

- Overconsumption of sugar leads to specific kidney problems that cause salt wasting.
- Chronic diseases such as hypothyroidism, adrenal insufficiency, and congestive heart failure can lead to hyponatremia (aka low blood sodium).
- Commonly prescribed medications such as diuretics, antidepressants, antipsychotics, and even some diabetes drugs leave us susceptible to salt depletion.
- Our java-junkie habits and our dependence on energy drinks, teas, and other caffeinated beverages put us at risk

for salt depletion because caffeine acts as a natural diuretic, flushing water and salt from our kidneys.

- Intense exercise causes us to lose considerable salt and water in sweat.
- And low-carb as well as intermittent (and especially prolonged) fasting diets cause massive losses of sodium and water from our kidneys and increase our need for salt.

I'm sure most of us can find ourselves somewhere on that list! Let's take a closer look at who should get less salt, who should get more, and how you can determine what level is best for you. Then, in the final chapter, we'll go over a basic program that will help everyone get the optimal amount of salt.

How Much Salt Do We Really Need?

While well-intentioned government departments and health authorities have focused primarily on the relationship between salt intake and blood pressure, they have largely overlooked the unintended consequences of not getting *enough* salt. As you've read throughout these pages, the dangers of salt depletion are far from trivial. These potential risks include an increase in heart rate, dehydration (which allows any sugar you eat to do more damage to your kidneys), cognitive impairment, bone fractures, food-borne illness (because salt inhibits the growth of bacteria in food), impaired oxygen and nutrient flow to the tissues, and even premature death. Not small risks! Plus, inadequate salt can make it harder for your body to activate fight-or-flight responses to cope with physiologically stressful situations such as gastrointestinal infections, blood loss, or a stroke or heart attack. And, as we just learned, a low salt intake could drive sugar addiction and even leave you vulnerable to drug addiction by sensitizing the dopamine receptors in your brain.

The optimal amount of salt can differ widely from person to person, depending on your unique situation. Here are a few important definitions to better understand terminology that will be discussed in this chapter.

Salt Set Point: This level of sodium intake maintains ideal health, longevity, and the best chances for survival of the species. This set point is determined by the brain and the body and, for most of us, seems to hover around 3 to 4 grams of sodium per day. The salt set point is an unconscious level of sodium intake, controlled by our body's salt thermostat, which may be higher or lower depending on the body's needs. (For example, if someone has salt-wasting kidneys, they may be consuming more sodium than a person with healthy kidneys because they are losing more—the body's need is driving this intake of salt instead of an "addictive" or hedonic drive.)

Sodium Balance: You reach this state when sodium in the urine matches sodium intake, taking into account nonkidney sodium losses, such as excretion in the feces and sweat. You are not losing salt from the body, nor are you retaining extra salt. Our sodium balance is maintained at the salt set point, which is a level of sodium intake around 3 to 4 grams per day for most people. Sodium balance in a healthy person can be maintained at sodium intakes as low as 230 to 300 milligrams of sodium per day—but this does not mean this is the optimal level of sodium intake for health and longevity. Rather, this indicates that body is in "crisis mode," a sodium-retaining pattern that causes an activation of salt-retaining hormones in order to maintain sodium balance at such a low intake.

Sodium Deficit: A simple way of knowing if someone has a sodium deficit (assuming they are healthy) is when they ingest sodium but none (or much less than what is consumed) is excreted in the urine.[1]

The Salt Thermostat: The salt set point is controlled by the salt thermostat of the body. The salt thermostat is a metaphor for a complex, interconnected set of sensors in your brain that work together to ensure the optimal sodium stores in the body, trying to avoid having to activate the salt-retaining hormones of your renin-angiotensin-aldosterone system. Your brain would really, *really* prefer that you simply eat more salt rather than having to hoard it or scavenge it from vulnerable parts of your body. These self-protective mechanisms help the body tightly control salt intake, causing you to crave salt when you need it. So when you crave salt, remember: that's your salt thermostat telling you that your body's sodium content is too low and that you need to eat more salt until you've reached the salt set point, the proper amount of sodium storage in the body.

Sodium balance can be maintained at the salt set point (consuming around 3,000 milligrams of sodium) but can also occur after about four to five days of salt restriction (generally after consuming around 300 milligrams of sodium or less per day). This is because it takes four to five days for your kidneys to slowly turn off the salt spilling out of them. However, after four to five days, your body finally shuts the sink off, so that you can maintain sodium balance by consuming as little as 300 milligrams of sodium per day (but that's only if you have healthy kidneys). Once you are in sodium balance, sodium excretion is slightly lower than intake because of nonkidney salt losses (such as from sweat and feces).[2] During sodium balance, if you take in more sodium than needed, most if not all sodium will be excreted. However, the ability of a healthy person to maintain sodium balance on a low-sodium diet (but not below 300 milligrams of sodium per day) does not mean that a low sodium intake is ideal or provides optimal health and longevity! In fact, being in sodium balance on a low-sodium diet requires the activation of certain rescue systems or salt-retaining hormones, which have been consistently found to induce harm. Salt-retaining hormones can harm the body's organs and may cause hypertension and other health consequences by causing enlargement as well as stiffening (fibrosis) of the heart and blood vessels.[3] This may be why low-salt diets are associated with greater cardiovascular risk and premature mortality. In general, a low salt intake places an individual at greater risk of salt deficit during sodium depletion. And there is no easy way of telling if someone has appropriate salt stores.

STOPPING SALT LOSS

Dieters are not the only people who struggle with salt wasting—even those with serious health concerns would likely benefit from adding high-quality salt sources. An elderly relative, who is now in her mideighties, was diagnosed with colon cancer around age forty. Luckily, her doctors caught it early enough and were able to remove the cancer—but they also had to remove most of her colon and give her a colostomy bag. The colon is vital for absorbing salt from the diet, and the kidneys are vital for reabsorbing the salt they filter out during their daily task of cleaning toxins out of your blood. As she began to age, her kidney function also declined, and her ability to hold on to the salt in her body also went down with age. All of this set her up to be a salt waster.

When she turned eighty-three, she kept feeling fatigued and dizzy and was constantly in the hospital for dehydration—and no one knew why. Luckily, I know a thing or two about salt! I told her how the colon is extremely important in absorbing salt from the diet, and how damage to the kidneys over the years can cause salt loss through urine—exactly the situation I suspected was happening. I told her that increasing her salt intake might help improve her dehydration—and, sure enough, it worked. Since she started enjoying more salt, she no longer feels as dizzy.

When you consume less sodium, your kidneys generally excrete less in order to maintain normal sodium balance and normal extracellular fluid volume. But if there is any problem with your kidneys' ability to retain sodium, you can become deficient in sodium rather quickly. (See the preceding story of my elderly family member; because of her damaged kidneys, she probably can't maintain sodium balance on a low-salt diet.) For example, during a hemorrhage, the kidneys almost immediately shut down sodium excretion to maintain normal blood volume.[4] And if your kidneys were unable to do this (for example, in patients who have tubulointerstitial damage in their kidneys from overconsuming refined sugar for decades), a bleeding event could be disastrous, particularly if the intake of salt is being restricted.

A phenomenal experiment published in the late 1950s looked at what would happen in someone who was in sodium balance while on a low-sodium diet if they experienced a sudden salt deficit, perhaps from gardening for hours on a hot day, a new prescription to control elevated blood pressure such as a diuretic, shock from trauma, burns, vomiting, or a bad bout of diarrhea. To simulate a sudden salt deficit, the patient was given a diuretic and lost 2,300 milligrams of sodium in the urine; the experiment found that after the patient ate salt again, there was no sodium excretion until the entire 2,300 milligrams of sodium was regained. This shows that the body can be in balance on a low-salt diet, but if something were to cause salt loss, the body would avidly retain salt until it reached sodium balance again. But if your kidneys are damaged and you are unable to hold on to extra salt, then you are in big trouble. In other words, when life throws you a salt-depleting curveball, the *last* thing you want is to be following the AHA advice to consume less than 1,500 milligrams of sodium per day. On the other hand, salt losses in people eating a normal-salt diet are much less likely to place them into salt deficit and cause subsequent harm. In essence, maintaining a normal sodium intake (3 to 4 grams) versus a low sodium intake (less than 2.3 grams) decreases your chances of becoming deficient if salt-depleting events occur. Experts believe we evolved with these sodium storage mechanisms to endure these salt-depleting events. The systems work best when we operate well above the minimal sodium intake (which, you'll recall, is just 300 milligrams per day) to maintain balance.[5]

In 1936, McCance performed what may be one of the most important studies to determine the ideal total body sodium content. Experimenting on himself, he was able to cause a net loss of 17.4 grams of sodium in his body, mostly through induced sweating.[6] McCance's urine became "virtually free of sodium" (less than 23 milligrams per day). When he began sodium repletion, consuming around 11.5 grams of sodium over the next two days, the urinary sodium excretion still remained at 23 milligrams per day—in essence, his body was still regaining all the salt he was consuming, indicating true salt deficit. The next day, he consumed 5,382 milligrams of sodium, bringing his three-day sodium intake to 16.836 grams (or 96.6 percent of what was lost) and, even then, only 368 milligrams of sodium was excreted in his urine. Remember, a normal sodium intake is about 3,400 milligrams per day, and we excrete all the sodium we take in every day under normal circumstances, so if you were to consume 5,382 milligrams of sodium, about 5,000 milligrams of sodium would be excreted in the urine, and the rest would come out in your sweat and stool for the day. But McCance's body was holding on to almost all of his sodium.

While this is only one example, his study suggests that just a 1-gram sodium loss from the body is problematic. If more than a 1-gram sodium loss were ideal for our body, then upon sodium repletion, we would continue to excrete sodium after reintroducing ample salt. But the body continues to hold on to all its ingested salt until it reaches within less than a few hundred milligrams of where it was prior to sodium depletion. We may be able to *survive* the loss of several dozen grams of sodium from the body, but a body deprived of salt will greedily hold on to replenished stores. We don't have much room for error when it comes to the optimal level of salt in our body.

In fact, studies show that sodium surplus seems to be what our biological system "drives" us to be in. Undoubtedly, someone in surplus would be much more likely to survive any type of sodium-depleting event (such as illness, diarrhea, infection, blood loss, or sweating). More importantly, sodium surplus keeps your salt-retaining hormones down, protecting your body from the resulting wear and tear on vital organs.

Sadly, governments and guidelines do not seem to give enough credence to the important fact that low-salt diets put stress on our bodies. Let's consider a few of the situations in which consuming a higher-salt diet could protect you from dire health concerns.

You May Need More Salt to Prevent Dehydration

You may be asking yourself, what typically causes dehydration? Does it happen often? What are the symptoms? We all say, "I feel dehydrated" when we are parched, but is that true dehydration? When you are parched, that is just one of the body's mechanisms to drive you to drink more water, and no one can say with certainty that a parched mouth indicates dehydration. Dehydration is typically caused by numerous factors, mainly by not consuming enough water, but it is also caused by exercise and not eating enough salt. The best measurement of dehydration is by looking at sodium levels in the blood; if they are high, then that is a good indication that you are dehydrated. Sodium

SYMPTOMS THAT MAY INDICATE A GREATER NEED FOR SALT[7]

Cold extremities

Dark urine

Decreased skin turgor (the skin remains "tented" when it is pinched)

Decreased urinary sodium excretion relative to intake

Decreased urine output

Dry axilla (armpit or underarm) and tongue

Poor capillary refill (takes longer than 2 seconds for the nail bed to return from white to pink after being pinched)

Postural tachycardia/dizziness/hypotension (occurs after rising from a seated or reclined position)

Salt cravings

Syncope (loss of consciousness from low blood pressure)

Thirst

levels increase in the blood for a few reasons, but mainly because with dehydration comes low blood volume, which increases the sodium concentration in the blood.

During states of dehydration, our kidneys step up their sodium reabsorption—an effect known as the dehydration reaction. Sodium helps manage how hydrated we are by controlling the movement of water into and out of our cells. When we're dehydrated, the sodium level in the blood increases because it's hard at work, drawing water out of the cells and into the blood, where it's needed. That's why highly concentrated sodium in the blood is almost always a sign of dehydration.[8] But that level of sodium isn't dangerous in and of itself—it's actually helping us!

A low sodium intake reduces urine volume,[9] which can reduce

RUNNING ON SALT

One family friend, who is a muscular middle-aged man and an avid runner, generally runs around ten miles a day during his training. Despite having maintained this regimen for years, he had never taken salt before or during his runs. After I counseled him on the potential benefits of salt prior to his long-distance runs, I asked him if he noticed any benefits. He said he noticed a definite difference on long runs, feeling less dehydration when he finished. He also noticed the benefits of salt dosing when running in warm temperatures (above 65 degrees). He noted that he is generally a "cold-weather runner." It makes sense that he finds cooler weather to be the optimal running temperature: we are less likely to overheat and lose salt and water at colder temperatures, because we're sweating less! Salt dosing prior to running may be particularly beneficial for those running in warmer/humid climates and those who are running at a fast pace or for a prolonged period.

our ability to clear metabolic wastes from the body and increases the risk of urinary tract infections. We rely on frequent urine flow in the urinary tract to get rid of bacteria; producing urine is our body's way of "flushing out the system." Eating a low-salt diet may also reduce the total amount of water in our body, leading to dehydration and problems with the cardiovascular and central nervous systems, thermoregulation, metabolic abnormalities, and performance issues (particularly in military and sports settings). This can increase the risk of fainting, vomiting, circulatory collapse, heatstroke, and even death.

You May Need More Salt to Help Manage Shock (Burns, Trauma, and Hemorrhage)

Salt helps the body withstand accidents and other kinds of traumatic events. Besides excessive bleeding (hemorrhage), we experience a loss of fluids in states of shock from burns or trauma.[10] This "loss" of body fluid happens without any water actually leaving the body, as injured regions draw fluid to speed the healing process, making that fluid unavailable to other areas. And since sodium is the main determinant of body fluid status, patients experiencing these forms of shock require greater amounts of salt. In fact, evidence suggests that a loss of salt is actually more dangerous than a loss of water,[11] because it decreases the body's ability to circulate blood around the body and reduces blood volume out of the heart more than water loss does. Salt depletion, even in untraumatized animals, can lead to a form of peripheral vascular collapse that looks like traumatic shock. This doesn't happen with water depletion.

You May Need More Salt to Counter Low Sodium Levels

Low sodium levels in the blood is called hyponatremia, and it's the most common electrolyte abnormality.[12] Approximately 65 percent of cases of hyponatremia in the ER are caused by gastrointestinal disorders.[13] When people seek medical treatment in an outpatient setting, 4 to 7 percent have hyponatremia; in the hospital, the rate can be as high as 42 percent (but is generally around 15 to 30 percent).[14] In the elderly, hyponatremia is over 31 *times as prevalent* as hypernatremia (high sodium levels in the blood)[15] and is associated with an increased risk of death, length of hospital stay, falls, rhabdomyolysis (rapid breakdown of muscle), bone fractures, and increased healthcare costs.[16] Even mild hyponatremia puts you at a higher risk of death due to cardiovascular events and increased risk of falls, bone fractures, and osteoporosis.[17]

Hyponatremia is also found in 18 percent of nursing home patients, and over 50 percent have at least one episode of hyponatremia a year. Nursing home patients have a *forty-three-fold higher* risk of being hospitalized with hyponatremia (with blood levels of sodium less than 135 mEq/L) and a sixteenfold higher risk of being admitted to the hospital with severe hyponatremia (with blood levels lower than 125 mEq/L) compared to patients in the community. One has to wonder if the low-salt meals that many nursing home patients are served as a matter of course are contributing to this pattern.

Medications such as selective serotonin reuptake inhibitors (SSRIs) can cause hyponatremia by triggering an oversecretion of antidiuretic hormone, leading to water retention. Small-cell lung cancer, malnutrition, and infections such as tuberculosis and pneumonia have the same effect.[18] Hyponatremia can also be caused by numerous other diseases: liver cirrhosis, pneumonia, and acquired immune deficiency syndrome (AIDS), to name just a few.[19] In addition to all the terrible symptoms that come along with hyponatremia—such as anorexia, cramping, nausea, vomiting, headache, irritability, disorientation, confusion, weakness, lethargy, and bone fractures—people with lower than 125 mEq/L can experience seizures, coma, permanent brain damage, respiratory arrest, and even death. One problem with chronic hyponatremia is that neurological symptoms may not be present until the serum sodium drops to 125 mEq/L or less, because of adaptive mechanisms in the brain—so someone could be walking around with low sodium levels in the blood and not even know it.[20]

Hypothyroidism, which becomes more common as people age, can cause salt-wasting kidney problems, as thyroid hormones are important in the functioning of Na-K-ATPase, which helps reabsorb salt at the kidney tubules.[21] Osmotic laxatives such as polyethylene glycol (for example, Miralax) may lead to salt wasting and volume depletion.[22] Hyponatremia can even be a complication of undergoing a colonoscopy, as the "bowel prep" induces massive diarrhea and salt loss.[23]

Many common medications that increase the risk of bleeding (such as nonsteroidal anti-inflammatory drugs [NSAIDs], aspirin, antiplatelets, and oral anticoagulants, to name just a few) also increase the risk of salt loss via blood. Indeed, it's been estimated that 16,500 people in the United States die every year from NSAID-induced gastrointestinal bleeding.[24] A higher-salt diet may have been able to help. Since it is not always apparent when someone has a gastrointestinal bleed, following the low-salt advice would not be advisable for someone taking medication that increases the risk of bleeding. (Sadly, many of these individuals probably never even knew they had a bleed until it was too late.)

You May Need More Salt When You Sweat

Fitness as a hobby has gone mainstream, and endurance training and competitions are becoming more popular than ever. Because they tend to be more conscious of their health, athletes are likely to follow recommendations to eat less salt. Unfortunately, these individuals may be at particular risk of salt depletion, not only from decreased consumption and increased losses of salt from sweat but also from overhydration with plain water. All of this adds up to low blood sodium levels.

Sweating helps the body maintain normal body temperature (aka thermoregulation) to prevent heatstroke—it's our body's way of cooling off. Having enough salt in the body to be able to adequately sweat is of vital importance in thermoregulation. The amount of sodium in our sweat generally ranges between 40 and 60 mEq/L, and we sweat out 1 to $1^1/_2$ liters per hour in moderate climates and 2 to 3 liters per hour in hot climates.[25] So, on average you will sweat out around 1,437 milligrams of sodium per hour when exercising in moderate climates and around 2,875 milligrams of sodium per hour when exercising in hot climates. Depending on exercise intensity and ambient temperature, you could easily lose more than an entire day's worth of salt intake in just one hour of exercise. In hot climates like India, you could lose up to 14,720 milligrams of sodium per day.[26] How would consuming just 1,500 milligrams of sodium per day (or even 2,300 milligrams of sodium) help you survive these conditions, let alone improve your health?

In one study by Mao and colleagues, one hour of soccer practice in temperature between 89.6°F and 98.6°F with 50 percent relative humidity caused players to lose 1,896 milligrams of sodium from sweating. One player actually lost almost 6,000 milligrams of sodium in sweat during the one-hour game. Importantly, soccer players also lost on average 52 micrograms of iodine in their sweat (and one player lost 100 micrograms); this amount of iodine loss is over one-third the recommended daily intake (150 micrograms per day). Almost half of the players were found to have a Grade 1 goiter, compared to 1 percent of the sedentary control subjects. It's very likely that because of continued iodine losses in sweat and not enough iodized salt intake, the players had developed goiters, which are a sign of severe thyroid problems. This happened despite the fact that the estimated iodine intake of soccer players, in general, met guideline recommendations (100 to 300 micrograms of iodine per day).[27] Bottom line: when you exercise, your body needs more salt and iodine than when you don't— and some people may need more than others.[28]

The average nonathletic adult excretes up to about 600 milligrams of sodium and about 22 micrograms of iodine in their average daily sweat. The average athlete, who sweats 3 to 5 liters per day, can lose between 111 and 185 micrograms of iodine in sweat, for a total iodine loss between 195 and 270 micrograms per day (when combined with loss from sweat, urine, and feces). Even consuming up to 340 micrograms of iodine per day, which is more than double the current recommended daily allowance (150 micrograms per day), could still lead to goiter and hypothyroidism in certain athletes. And it's not just athletes: iodine losses during the summer correlate with an increased prevalence of goiter among school-age children.[29] (Especially during the hotter months, you can ensure that your family gets sufficient iodine by seeking out more foods rich in iodine, such as seaweed, cranberries, and yogurt.)

Goiters aren't the only risk. Depletion of body sodium can lead to symptoms comparable to overtraining syndrome, even before we can detect lower levels of sodium in the blood. Salt depletion can cause the body to work harder than normal, pushing you into training overload prematurely. Your physical strength starts to falter and your sympathetic nervous system gets so exhausted that your blood pressure drops and you're at risk of fainting. Part of the reason sodium depletion may lead to impaired muscular strength and energy metabolism is that it raises the acidity of our cells.[30]

People who aren't in the best shape may take longer to finish athletic competitions, and that extended time exercising may increase risk of hyponatremia.[31] The consequences of excessive losses of salt (and other minerals) in sweat during exercise can include dehydration, tremors, muscular weakness, and even cardiac arrhythmias.[32] In one report, a reduced sodium intake during high-intensity exercise increased cramps and muscle fatigue; reduced endurance performance; and caused general fatigue, joint pain, sleeping disorders, circulatory impairments, and distinct thirst. But these symptoms were vastly improved when people increased their sodium intake—even when they worked out harder, their symptoms of overtraining were eliminated.[33]

The "thirst" that we experience during bouts of exercise, particularly among endurance athletes, may actually be for the replacement of salt, not water. If we increase salt intake, we may find we have less "thirst."[34] Tap water has a sodium content of only 1 to 3 mmol/L,[35] whereas sweat contains 20 to 80 mmol of sodium per liter. Basically, your sweat is seven to eighty times as concentrated in sodium as tap water—so you should be hydrating with something that contains much more salt than just plain tap water.

Athletes who struggle with arthritis could experience relief with extra salt. Here's why: cartilage cells (chondrocytes) contain sodium/hydrogen (Na/H)-antiporter systems. When you don't have enough sodium in your cartilage cells, acid (hydrogen, H+) can build up. And that's not good for your cartilage or your joints. In osteoarthritis and rheumatoid arthritis, the excess fluid that surrounds inflamed cartilage cells can dilute the sodium level in those areas, which may lead to further pain.[36] Thus, low-salt diets may worsen cartilage health in both those with and without autoimmune diseases, decreasing their ability to protect joints and increasing joint pain, especially during exercise. Thus, low-salt diets can be a triple whammy for runners—they

---

BEAT THE HEAT

The day David Harris, a fit, athletic, young dad of two, ran his first marathon in Boston, the temperature hit about 90 degrees. He had prepared the best he could from an exercise standpoint, doing many long runs in preparation. But that day, in the heat, he found that he started cramping up around mile 18. After the race, David talked with me about his muscle cramps and I suggested that he take a salt supplement prior to and during races. Since that day, he's taken salt tabs during longer training rides and runs, as well as at each of his races, which now include two Ironmans, two half Ironmans, two marathons, and a half marathon. In all of those events, the salt supplements helped him tremendously—he has not cramped up at all since.

lose salt from their sweat, from the fluid surrounding their cartilage cells, and even from within the cartilage cells themselves.

What to Do for Exercise

The answer is simple: Consume more salt before and during exercise. It may help your body cool off faster.[37] Adding 2,300 milligrams of sodium (1 teaspoon of salt) per liter of water has been found to reduce total fluid loss during exercise.[38] In the largest field-based study, the prevalence of hyponatremia in triathlon finishers was 18 percent, most likely caused by overhydration.[39] But that doesn't mean you can or should prevent hyponatremia by drinking less water. Rather, drink the same amount, but add the appropriate level of salt to whatever liquids you are drinking.

I find that taking organic garlic salt straight out of the teaspoon is more palatable than using pure table salt, with or without water. A good dose of salt (if working out in moderate climates) is $1/2$ teaspoon of table salt (a little bit more if using garlic salt). This provides about 1,150 milligrams of sodium and should cover most of your salt losses during the first hour of your workout. Take this prophylactic dose of salt about thirty minutes prior to your workout, with an additional $1/2$ teaspoon of salt for every hour thereafter, and you may see significant gains in your performance. Dumping the salt out onto a teaspoon and consuming it dry (and then rinsing out the mouth with some water) is much more pleasant than dumping $1/2$ teaspoon of salt into a liter of water and consuming it (as the latter tastes like you are literally drinking sweat; it's rather nauseating!). Also, diluting salt in a mixture of lemon, lime, and orange juice is quite pleasant. Sometimes I will even grab a teaspoon or more of soy sauce or guzzle down some pickle juice before my workouts, in order to up my salt status.

If you are on a long endurance run, you may want to carry a small pouch of salt along with a plastic $1/2$-teaspoon measuring spoon. After each hour of exercise, simply scoop out the dose of salt recommended in the list "Recommendations for Salt Dosing Prior to and During

Exercise" (see page 136), based on ambient temperature, and consume. Replacing the amount of salt that is lost through sweat helps your body's thirst mechanism. Your body will tell you how much water to drink, and it will do this more accurately, when you consume the appropriate amount of salt—which will also reduce your risk of overhydration.

Dosing yourself with salt prior to and during exercise should also help your body cool off faster and improve blood circulation (and hence nutrient/oxygen delivery to the tissues) and water retention (enhancing body hydration status), and better your overall performance (improved blood flow and increased detoxification of acid buildup in tissues), all while reducing your risk of cramping and fatigue. The first list that follows shows some benefits you may enjoy after adding salt prior to and during your workout regimen. The two lists that follow that provide recommendations for salt intake prior to and during exercise.

POSSIBLE BENEFITS OF DOSING YOURSELF WITH SALT PRIOR TO AND DURING EXERCISE

Less thirst (helps to quench "thirst," so less water consumed and less risk for overhydration hyponatremia)

Greater exercise capacity (greater ability to train longer due to enhanced body cooling, improved circulation and tissue oxygenation/blood flow [better "pump"], improved body hydration, decreased tissue acidosis/hyponatremia, and improved cartilage health)

Improved performance

Improved muscle gains

Decreased risk of hyponatremia (elevated blood sodium levels lead to decreased risk for arrhythmias, cramps, and fatigue)

Decreased risk of iodine deficiency (if using iodized salt)

Improved kidney function (improving the ability to excrete more water, which decreases the risk of dilutional hyponatremia, making the kidneys less sensitive to the effects of antidiuretic hormone [reducing the risk of overretention of water and subsequent hyponatremia])[40]

**HOW TO CONSUME YOUR DOSE OF SALT
PRIOR TO AND DURING EXERCISE**

Measure out your dose of salt using a teaspoon and consume dry, then rinse your mouth out with water (or pickle juice)

Eat three large dill pickles (or five large olives) washed down with some pickle/olive juice

Dissolve a chicken bouillon cube(s) in warm water and consume

Dissolve $1/2$ teaspoon of salt in 1 liter of water (tastes like sweat, not recommended)

Dissolve salt in a mixture of lemon/lime/orange juice or lemonade and consume (preferred method). If you are an avid exerciser, I recommend that you use a salt that also contains iodine, such as Redmond Real Salt, but iodized table salt will also work.

**RECOMMENDATIONS FOR SALT DOSING
PRIOR TO AND DURING EXERCISE**

Exercising in moderate climates (below 80°F)

Consume $1/2$ teaspoon of salt prior to exercise and every hour thereafter

Exercising in hot climates (80°F to 89°F)

Consume $1/2$ to 1 teaspoon of salt prior to exercise and every hour thereafter

Exercising in very hot climates (90°F or above)

Consume 1 to 2 teaspoons of salt prior to exercise and every hour thereafter

*These are only estimates. The salt dose will depend on how much you sweat, which is determined by genetics, clothing, level of exercise intensity, and ambient temperature. And, of course, always get your doctor's approval first before changing any of your diet or lifestyle habits.

Note: Patients who are exercising or performing activities that lead to excessive sweating and who are also on salt-depleting medications such as diuretics (such as hydrochlorothiazide or furosemide), angiotensin-converting enzyme inhibitors (such as ramipril or lisinopril), or mineralocorticoid receptor antagonists (such as spironolactone or eplerenone) may need to use even more salt than what has been recommended in the preceding list "Recommendations for Salt Dosing Prior to and During Exercise."

MORE SALT WHEN IN THE SAUNA

While the health benefits of heat and sweating from saunas, sun baths, tanning beds, and Jacuzzis have been debated for years, one issue beyond debate is the increased risk of tissue sodium depletion. It may also be a good idea to consume salt prior to thermal-induced dehydration. Follow the salt dose recommendations in the "Recommendations for Salt Dosing Prior to and During Exercise" list on page 136 before hitting the sauna.

You May Need More Salt When Pregnant or Lactating

Earlier in the book, I talked about how lower salt intake has a proven link with lower reproductive success. Indeed, a low-salt diet seems to act like a natural contraceptive in both men and women, causing reduced sex drive; reduced likelihood of getting pregnant; reduced litter size (in animals) and weight of infants; and increased erectile dysfunction, fatigue, sleep problems, and age at which women become fertile.[41] We can see the importance of salt in fertility in the low incidence of pregnancy among the low-salt-eating Yanomamo Indians, who average only one live birth every four to six years, despite being sexually active and not using contraception.[42] Women with congenital adrenal hyperplasia (specifically those with salt-wasting nephropathies) have a decreased fertility and childbirth rate.[43]

A mother's salt status not only determines her ability to get pregnant but may control the future health of her infants. Because salt is so important for numerous functions in the body, a depletion of salt from either a lack of dietary intake (following the low-salt recommendations) or salt loss (think of nausea and vomiting during pregnancy) not only may worsen the health of the mother but can impair the health of the growing child even into adulthood. Pregnancy and lactation place increased nutritional demands on the mother in order to supply the baby with enough nutrients for proper growth and development[44]—and salt is one of those nutrients. Salt restriction in pregnant or lactating mothers seems to increase the vulnerability of their children to multiple hazardous outcomes.

For example, in animals, low salt intake during pregnancy and/or lactation leads to increased fat mass, insulin resistance, and raised levels of "bad" cholesterol and triglycerides in the offspring, which may carry over into adulthood.[45] More worrisome is that a low-salt diet in pregnancy has also been found to cause hypertension and kidney disease in adult offspring.[46] All of this suggests that low salt intake during pregnancy may program our children to develop abnormal lipids, diabetes, obesity, hypertension, and chronic kidney disease—the very diseases we believe a low-salt diet will prevent!

Sadly, the increased physiological need for salt during pregnancy conflicts with population-wide low-salt advice, which has been entrenched into our minds by government and health agencies. The American Heart Association, for example, recommends that all Americans reduce their daily sodium intake to less than 1,500 milligrams, and women of childbearing years or who are pregnant or lactating do not appear to be exempt from this advice. Even the World Health Organization (WHO) recommends that pregnant and lactating women restrict their sodium intake to less than 2 grams per day.[47] But these recommendations may have unintended consequences. Health agencies and government bodies seem to have forgotten that dietary iodine requirements increase by 50 percent or more during pregnancy and lactation,[48] and that iodized salt has been an important way to prevent iodine deficiency for decades. Indeed, the WHO recommends that pregnant and lactating women consume 250 micrograms of iodine per day.[49] However, even if all maternal dietary salt intake during pregnancy/lactation comes from iodized salt, the Recommended Nutrient Intake (RNI) for iodine (250 micrograms per day) will still not be met by following these low-salt recommendations! And we can't assume that pregnant and lactating women know to eat enough high-iodine foods every day to make up the difference.

Considering that iodine deficiency during pregnancy is the leading cause of mental retardation, health agencies may want to rethink their low-salt advice during this critical time in human development. An iodine deficiency in pregnancy or lactation can also lead to impaired motor function and growth as well as hypothyroidism, and even perinatal and infant death.[50] Moreover, national data indicates that weaning babies may not have adequate iodine intake and thus may benefit from a greater iodized salt intake.[51]

Indeed, what we currently think is an "adequate" iodine intake in pregnancy may actually be insufficient, as data suggests that over 36 percent of pregnant women develop hypothyroidism (or thyroid insufficiency), even among pregnant women with "adequate" iodine status in the first trimester.[52] Importantly, iodine deficiency is still a significant health problem worldwide that affects both industrialized and developing nations, with fifty-four countries still considered iodine deficient.[53] This is perhaps why the Council for Responsible Nutrition (CRN) recently recommended that dietary supplements should include at least 150 micrograms of iodine in all supplements intended for pregnant and lactating women in the United States.[54] But until then, telling pregnant and lactating women to consciously restrict their salt intake increases their risk for iodine deficiency and may be a decidedly harmful recommendation.

One myth that persists is that too much salt during pregnancy can lead to preeclampsia, a dangerous condition characterized by hypertension that can endanger both mother and child and lead to premature birth, among other complications. Over fifty years ago, a study published in the *Lancet* of more than two thousand pregnant women found that a low-salt diet, as compared to a high-salt diet, caused more miscarriages, premature babies (born prior to 34 weeks gestation), stillbirths, perinatal and neonatal deaths, edema, preeclampsia (previously known as toxemia), and bleeding.[55] And since there was less preeclampsia in those on the high-salt diet, it was decided later that cases of preeclampsia would be treated with extra dietary salt. Between the end of May and the end of September 1957, twenty-eight women were diagnosed with what was then known as "toxemia of pregnancy." Eight were not given extra salt, while the other twenty were advised to ingest more dietary salt. All of the twenty women treated with extra salt improved, and all gave birth to healthy, full-term babies. An account of the study said, "the larger the dose of salt taken, the quicker and more complete was the recovery. The extra dose of salt had to be taken up to the time of delivery; otherwise the symptoms of toxemia recurred." In other words, giving more salt *treated* preeclampsia rather than causing or worsening it (a common misconception). Consider this account from the researcher (from the study published in the *Lancet*):

> Sixteen patients were advised to measure out each morning four heaped teaspoonfuls of table salt and to see that by night they had taken all of it. It was calculated that they took about *200–300 grams of salt daily* [emphasis added]. The larger the amount taken the quicker was the recovery. They found it easiest to take the bulk of this salt in orange-juice, lemonade, or lime-juice, the remainder being put on their food. They were visited daily until all symptoms had disappeared. All of them recovered completely and continued well on at least three heaped teaspoonfuls of table salt a day. None of them had an infarcted placenta, and all gave birth to live full-term infants.[56]

In contrast, certain side effects were also noted in the eight women who followed salt restriction, such as:

severe backache, some [complained] of irritation of the skin of arms, legs, or abdomen, and some of weariness and stiffness in the limbs. Others complained of falling because their legs suddenly gave way under them. Sometimes this was so severe that they were afraid of going out of their houses or of crossing the road, in case they fell. These symptoms did not develop in the group given salt, and if they were present at the first examination they disappeared as soon as the women took more salt.[57]

In other words, low-salt diets in pregnancy seem to lead to muscle weakness, particularly in the legs, which was treated by giving more salt. The authors concluded that extra salt in the diet seemed to be "essential for the health of a pregnant woman, her fetus, and the placenta."[58] Because of the risks involved, ethics boards would not likely approve this kind of study today. With these kinds of results in only two small randomized controlled trials testing a low-salt versus a normal-salt diet in just a few hundred pregnant women, we may want to give strong reconsideration to the practice of recommending low-salt diets in pregnant women.[59]

Another paper described the experience of a pregnant woman with elevated blood pressure and evidence of low aldosterone levels who was given 20 grams of salt per day, which led to a decrease in systolic and diastolic blood pressure of 16 and 12 mmHg, respectively. The authors concluded that low blood volume during pregnancy might be due to a reduced ability to produce aldosterone and that pregnant women would probably benefit from salt supplementation.[60] Another study confirmed these findings, saying they "support the importance of salt in normal pregnancy, a critical issue given the passionate campaigns to lower salt intake in the general population." The researchers suggested that salt could be a "cheap and easy intervention," particularly in areas with lower resources, to help avoid dangerous pregnancy conditions such as preeclampsia.[61] The possible harms of a low-salt diet in pregnancy or those trying to become pregnant are summarized in the list that follows.

Consuming more salt may even help prevent pregnant women with normal blood pressure from transitioning into hypertension/preeclampsia, as low plasma volume is a risk factor for developing hypertension in these women.[62] In fact, blood volume has consistently been found to be reduced in preeclampsia, and its improvement may be why salt is so helpful for treating preeclampsia in pregnancy.[63]

THE POSSIBLE HARMS OF A LOW-SALT DIET IN PREGNANCY OR THOSE TRYING TO BECOME PREGNANT

Reduced chance of becoming pregnant

Increased chance of a miscarriage

Increased risk of premature delivery

Increased risk of infant mortality

Increased risk of bleeding in the mother

Increased risk of preeclampsia

Increased risk of low-birth-weight babies who will become chronic salt cravers/addicts with higher risk of obesity, insulin resistance, hypertension, and compromised kidney function

You May Need More Salt for Energy and Muscle Health

One side effect of low-salt diets that is seen in almost every population is reduced energy and increased fatigue. Consider the findings of the Trial of Antihypertensive Interventions and Management (TAIM), a multicenter, randomized, placebo-controlled clinical trial that evaluated nine different combinations of diet and medications for the treatment of mild hypertension.[64] The average change in sodium intake in the TAIM Study was from 3,128 milligrams per day at baseline down to 2,484 milligrams per day after six months. This reduction of over 600 milligrams per day was found to cause worsening fatigue, sleep disturbances, and erectile dysfunction.[65] In other words, salt restriction drastically reduces the quality of life. Moreover, as much as they tried, only 25 percent of people were able to reduce their sodium intake to below 1,610 milligrams per day.[66] Compared with the control group, twice the number of people on the low-sodium diet complained of fatigue, with more than one out of three patients having an increase in fatigue symptoms.[67]

Among patients with chronic fatigue syndrome, 61 percent have reported that they "usually or always tried to avoid salt and salty foods,"[68] presumably because they believe it is healthy for them to do so. But this may be a decidedly unhealthy decision.[69] Low-salt diets may lead to weaker muscles and increase or worsen chronic fatigue syndrome, and may be particularly harmful in people with conditions that share chronic fatigue syndrome's symptoms of hypotension, dizziness, light-headedness, and syncope (temporary loss of consciousness), such as Parkinson's disease.[70]

If you have any of these symptoms or conditions but are trying to combat them with exercise, low-salt diets may increase the likelihood of injuries during workouts, cause longer recovery periods, and decrease your muscle gains. Additionally, side effects from certain medications could be made worse. For example, muscle pain is a common side effect of statins, and low-salt diets may predispose to this side effect, further preventing people from exercising on statins and increasing the risk of weight gain.

You Need More Salt When High-Sugar Diets Lead to Salt Wasting

Not only do high glucose levels in the blood deplete the body of sodium through increased excretion; they can also lower the blood sodium level overall. High glucose in the blood is known to reduce blood sodium levels as it pulls water out of the cells and into the blood.[71] Those with poorly controlled diabetes and high levels of sugar in their blood may be at risk of sodium depletion as high glucose levels can cause this osmotic diuresis, as well as salt wasting and hyponatremia.[72] A list follows that covers the twenty-two ways sugar causes salt depletion.

All of this suggests that once glucose levels are chronically elevated, giving someone more salt may actually improve health—and may even be lifesaving. In one study of patients with insulin resistance, researchers found that giving around 6,000 milligrams of sodium per day as compared to 3,000 milligrams of sodium per day ameliorated their insulin resistance.[73] With over 50 percent of adults in the United States now considered diabetic or prediabetic, low-salt diets may be causing harm to over half the adult population.[74]

TWENTY-TWO WAYS SUGAR CAUSES SALT DEPLETION

1. **Sugar** → damages intestinal cells → celiac disease/Crohn's disease/ulcerative colitis → decreased absorption of salt via the intestines[75]

2. **Sugar** → fructose malabsorption → irritable bowel syndrome → diarrhea → increased salt excretion[76]

3. **Sugar** → *Candida albicans* → irritable bowel syndrome → diarrhea → salt wasting from gastrointestinal tract[77]

4. **Sugar** → damages the reabsorptive capacity of the kidneys (tubulointerstitial damage) → salt-wasting kidneys[78]

5. **Sugar** → damages kidneys → reduced glomerular filtration rate → preferential retention of water → low sodium and chloride levels in the blood[79]

6. **Sugar** → damages the juxtaglomerular cells (atrophy of the juxtaglomerular apparatus) and kidney tubules → decreased renin production (low-renin hypertension) → decreased aldosterone (and decreased response of the kidney tubules to aldosterone) → increased sodium excretion → sodium wasting[80]

7. **Sugar** → diabetic dysautonomia (malfunction of the autonomic nervous system) → decreased conversion of pro-renin to renin by the kidney → low renin → low aldosterone → sodium wasting[81]

8. **Sugar** → damages the heart → congestive heart failure → preferential retention of water to maintain cardiac output → risk of low blood levels of sodium and chloride[82]

9. **Sugar** → damages the liver → fatty liver → liver cirrhosis → overretention of water → low blood levels of sodium and chloride[83]

10. **Sugar** → increases blood glucose levels → increased need for water in the blood to prevent hyperglycemia → low blood levels of sodium and chloride[84]

11. **Sugar** → hyperglycemia → osmotic diuresis (polyuria/natriuresis) → hypovolemic hyponatremia (sodium elimination via urine when glucose levels are uncontrolled)[85] (For every 100 mg/dL increase in plasma glucose above 150 mg/dL, serum sodium will drop by approximately 2.4 mEq/L.[86] Patients with diabetes who have uncontrolled glucose levels have a higher risk for hyponatremia.)[87]

12. **Sugar** → diabetic ketoacidosis → ketones promote sodium elimination → renal sodium wasting[88]

13. **Sugar** → diabetes → diabetic medications (sodium-glucose cotransporter 2 [SGLT2] inhibitors, acarbose, metformin, sulfonylureas) → increased sodium elimination and/or risk of hyponatremia (from reduced insulin levels, reduced absorption and increased elimination of sodium, increased secretion of antidiuretic hormone)[89]

14. **Sugar** → diabetes → reabsorption of hypotonic fluids due to delayed gastric emptying → low blood levels of sodium and chloride[90]

15. **Sugar** → hypertension → antihypertensive medications (many of which deplete sodium such as diuretics, beta-blockers, ACE inhibitors, mineralocorticoid receptor antagonists) → risk of hyponatremia

16. **Sugar** → obesity → increase in exercise to try to lose/maintain weight → salt wasting from sweat → salt depletion

17. **Sugar** → inflammation, oxidative stress, cellular damage, high insulin levels → cancer → low sodium levels in the blood[91] → certain anticancer medications (cisplatin) → salt-wasting nephropathy[92]

18. **Sugar** → obesity → bariatric surgery → reduced absorption of salt → risk of salt depletion[93]

19. **Sugar** → *Candida albicans* → proteins in *Candida albicans* can bind to thyroxine → allergic response to *Candida albicans* cross-reacts with thyroxine → autoimmune thyroiditis → hypothyroidism → salt depletion[94]

20. **Sugar** → *Candida albicans* → reduced lactase activity in the small intestine → lactose intolerance → diarrhea → increased salt excretion[95] (Importantly, sugar compounds are required for *Candida* to bind to intestinal mucosal membranes, and thus sugar is required for *Candida* to cause lactose intolerance.)[96]

21. **Sugar** → *Candida albicans* → immunologic response → cross-allergy to gluten → celiac disease → damage to intestinal microvilli → reduced salt absorption[97]

22. **Sugar** → one-kidney renal artery stenosis → renal ischemia → high renin → high angiotensin-II (leads to high antidiuretic hormone [ADH]) → thirst and water retention → hyponatremia → increased blood pressure → pressure natriuresis through the normal kidney → volume depletion → further ADH release → hyponatremic-hypertensive syndrome[98]

You May Need More Salt for Kidney Disease

As we age, our levels of renin and aldosterone are reduced, and with them, our kidneys' ability to retain salt, increasing our risk of salt deficit.[99] People with chronic renal insufficiency—kidneys that do not function at their optimal level—cannot maintain the optimal level of sodium in their body, even when they follow a normal or average sodium intake. One study found deficits in excess of 5,750 to 6,900 milligrams of sodium after only three or four days when sodium intake was reduced to 690 to 920 milligrams of sodium per day.

One sign that you may have salt-wasting kidney disease is if more sodium comes out in your urine than the amount you are eating. If you have salt-wasting kidney disease, you may require more than 6 to 7 grams of sodium per day to maintain stable kidney function. If you cut your sodium to 1,610 to 2,300 milligrams of sodium per day, you could promptly become severely ill because of low blood volume and compromised kidney function.[100] In essence, following the low-salt advice (less than 2,300 milligrams of sodium per day) may lead to kidney failure, circulatory collapse, and even death in patients with salt-wasting kidney disease. People who have chronically elevated aldosterone levels when they eat a normal salt intake, or up to tenfold higher aldosterone levels when you're on a low-sodium diet, may be showing signs of salt-wasting kidney disease.

The sodium pumps of the kidney not only help to remove potassium but also function to reabsorb sodium. Structural damage or changes to the kidneys can reduce the sodium pumps' ability to absorb sodium and excrete potassium. If this is the case, inappropriately high blood potassium can indicate damage to the sodium pumps and can be easier to detect than sodium loss via the kidney.[101]

As our kidneys age, their ability to excrete water decreases, predisposing the elderly to hyponatremia.[102] Additionally, as we age, the risk of metabolic acidosis increases, which is considered a side effect of eating a Western diet.[103] The extra acid (hydrogen ions) then needs to be secreted via the urine, increasing the risk of renal tubular acidosis and decreasing the kidneys' ability to retain sodium.[104] The kidneys of patients with hypertension may overretain water or reabsorb insufficient amounts of salt (sodium chloride) or both.[105] This means that patients with hypertension or certain kidney diseases may need more salt, to balance not only the high amounts of retained water but also the loss of salt via the kidneys.

A reduction in the intake of sodium has been found to impair kidney function and reduce kidney plasma flow and filtration rate.[106] Even in uncomplicated hypertension, low-salt diets can cause marked decreases in serum sodium and chloride[107] and even induce shock due to sudden falls in blood pressure.[108] In people whose kidney function has taken a hit and who also have low blood pressure, increasing their intake of salt can show immediate improvements in symptoms of shock.[109] One group of authors concluded that the benefits of low-salt diets for hypertension were unproven but warned that "strict low sodium diets are unpalatable, require extensive environmental and psychological adjustments, and carry the occasional risks of inanition and—particularly in the presence of renal damage—of collapse, uremia and even death."[110]

Low-salt diets can also reduce our kidneys' filtration rate, which can increase our body's retention of nitrogen—and may even lead to death in patients with uremia, a condition of fluid, hormone, and electrolyte imbalance in which toxic by-products build up in the blood. In fact, one group of authors noted the harms of salt deprivation: "significant nitrogen retention, and death in uremia has been reported in at least two hypertensive patients on this regimen."[111] Many commonly prescribed medications, including those that lower heart rate (atenolol, for example) or prevent stroke in patients with atrial fibrillation (such as dabigatran) are cleared by the kidneys. If individuals start lowering their salt intake while on medications that are cleared by the kidneys, this could reduce that clearance, increasing the concentration of these drugs in the blood and hence increasing the risk for serious side effects (and even possibly death). Of course, low-salt guidelines do not make any mention of this important side effect to the kidneys upon sodium restriction, so clinicians and patients are generally unaware of this risk.

Our kidneys' ability to dilute our urine decreases as we progress further into kidney disease.[112] And since patients with chronic kidney disease have a reduction in kidney filtration rate, we start to retain water, increasing the risk of both dangerously increased blood volume and hyponatremia. As the kidneys' primary function is to reabsorb all sodium that gets filtered, a reduction in glomerular filtration does not seem to cause sodium retention (as we reabsorb about 99 percent of the sodium that is filtered by the kidneys; the other 1 percent comes from our diet). Even if there is a true overretention of sodium by the kidneys, the liver can signal the intestine to reduce sodium absorption, and both the liver and gastrointestinal systems can signal the kidneys to reabsorb less sodium.[113] Additionally, the body can shunt extra salt into the skin and organs and possibly even into the cartilage/bone.[114] All of these secondary mechanisms suggest that the human body is well adapted to handle salt overload—but not salt deficit.

Sodium restriction is particularly harmful in chronic kidney disease because hyponatremia is extremely common (13.5 percent). In fact, more than one out of four chronic kidney disease patients (26 percent) will experience at least one episode of hyponatremia during a five-year period, whereas the rate of hypernatremia is less than one in fourteen people (7 percent). The prevalence of hyponatremia seems to go down slightly with advancing kidney disease but is still much more prevalent than hypernatremia. Hyponatremia is twenty to thirty times as prevalent as hypernatremia in chronic kidney disease stages 1 and 2, five to seven times as prevalent in stage 3, and about four times as prevalent in stages 4 and 5.[115]

Interestingly, the impact of hyponatremia on mortality has a similar magnitude no matter what stage of chronic kidney disease, whereas the magnitude of mortality with hypernatremia is less pronounced when it becomes more prevalent (during later stages of kidney disease). This indicates that while high sodium levels in the blood may become slightly more prevalent in later stages of kidney disease (stages 4 and 5), they are not as harmful. This may be because the body has ample time to adapt to the high blood sodium levels, which does not seem to occur with low sodium levels in the blood.[116]

In one study, hyponatremia and hypernatremia both predicted increased mortality, with the lowest risk of mortality found at a serum sodium level of 140 to 144 mEq/L.[117] Other experts have defined the optimal range of blood sodium as between 139 and 143 mEq/L.[118] If your blood sodium level is not in this optimal range, you may need to eat more (or less) salt. The risks of dying with serum sodium levels greater than 145 mEq/L (hypernatremia) and between 130 and 135.9 mEq/L (hyponatremia) do not seem to significantly differ from one another in patients with chronic kidney disease. However, once blood sodium levels fall below 130 mEq/L, the risk of death is almost twofold compared to just 1.3-fold with a blood sodium level greater than 145 mEq/L).

In summary, hyponatremia is extremely common in chronic kidney disease, especially when compared to hypernatremia. Restricting sodium in patients with chronic kidney disease is not necessarily a good idea and may lead to adverse health outcomes. If anything, patients with chronic kidney disease may benefit from eating more salt. Even hemodialysis patients (who generally lack an ability to excrete salt in between dialysis sessions) may actually benefit from eating more salt, as hyponatremia increases the risk of mortality in these patients as well.[119] Low dietary sodium intake is also associated with an increase in the risk of death in peritoneal dialysis,[120] and hyponatremia is a complication in peritoneal dialysis.[121]

Low-salt diets may also make sugar more harmful to the kidneys, as they can lead to dehydration, which activates the "polyol pathway" in the kidneys that causes us to form more fructose from glucose, metabolize fructose more quickly, and increases our oxidative stress and damage to our kidneys.[122] And, again, all of this can lead to salt-wasting kidneys. In essence, if you choose a low salt intake on top of a high-sugar diet, you have the perfect formula for causing kidneys that can no longer hold on to salt.[123] That's why low-salt diets are potentially extremely harmful in those consuming diets high in sugar, especially in patients with diabetes.[124]

You May Need More Salt if You Have Inflammatory Bowel Disease

The surgical removal of the small intestine can lead to intestinal failure, "short bowel syndrome," and reduce a person's ability to absorb salt.[125] However, the intestine can also fail because of inflammation, ischemia, or motility disorders. The primary task of the colon, besides moving fecal material out of the body, is to absorb salt and water. Patients with inflammatory bowel disease (Crohn's and ulcerative colitis) have significant problems absorbing salt in the intestine and colon, respectively, which leads to excreting more salt and lower blood sodium levels, even in moments of remission.[126] People who have had part of their colon removed (during treatment for colon cancer, for example) are also at risk of developing sodium and water depletion.[127] In fact, any damage to the intestinal mucosa, such as celiac disease, will reduce the absorption of salt—and increase the risks of following a low-salt diet.

LOW-CARB CRAMPS CURED

A general practitioner friend of mine, David Unwin, MD, recently began struggling with a painful affliction. He'd been following a low-carb eating plan for some time when he started developing painful and embarrassing leg cramps that could make him cry out without warning. These cramps would come upon him at the most inconvenient moments— such as when he was in consultation with a patient! The cramps likely resulted from the low-carb diet he'd begun to follow. All of these painful, annoying, inconvenient symptoms disappeared as soon as he added extra salt to his diet.

You May Need More Salt on Low-Carbohydrate Diets

Patients eating low-carbohydrate diets will need more salt (especially during the first two weeks of the diet) compared to someone who has higher levels of insulin (someone eating over 50 grams of carbohydrates per day). Higher levels of ketones, greater release of glucagon, and lower levels of insulin, all of which occur on a low-carb diet, increase our excretion of sodium.[128]

When dietary carbohydrate is restricted to 50 grams per day, the same excretion of sodium that occurs during starvation occurs with this level of carb restriction.[129] In one study of normal healthy patients, despite eating more than 100 grams of protein and 1,500 to 2,000 calories per day, their elimination of carbohydrates caused a significant sodium depletion of about 4.7 to 5.6 grams in just three days. The sodium depletion that was previously attributed to the lack of calories during fasting turned out to be the result of carbohydrate restriction.[130] Another study of obese subjects showed that 4,266 milligrams of sodium was depleted from the body in just seven days on a low-carbohydrate (40 grams per day) diet.[131] Eliminating carbohydrate intake in healthy patients, down to 0 grams per day (as found in one fasting/starvation study) for ten days was found to deplete 18.72 grams of sodium from the body, just from losses via the urine.[132] In another study of forty obese patients, people lost an average of 8 to 19 grams of sodium over ten days.[133] Another fasting study of seven obese females found that they went through their sodium excretion in five- to six-day cycles, losing between 18.6 and 57.3 grams of sodium over a period of thirty days.[134] It's clear that low-carbohydrate diets (as well as prolonged fasting) can cause a dramatic reduction in total body sodium content (and hence a greater risk of sodium deficit). The losses of sodium in the urine on low-carb diets seem to dissipate after about two weeks as the body makes its adjustment. However, compared to when they followed a previous diet that was higher in carbohydrates, individuals following low-carb diets keep losing more salt in the urine because of the reduction in insulin levels. They may experience symptoms such as dizziness, fatigue, and carb cravings, which could be greatly improved by upping their salt intake.

ADDING SALT TO A LOW-CARB DIET

Most patients who start a low-carbohydrate diet (less than 50 grams of carbohydrates per day) will lose between 4 and 8 grams of sodium in ten days, but some may lose up to 20 grams during this time. That's why it's a good idea to increase your sodium intake by at least 1 gram per day for the first two weeks of a low-carbohydrate diet or by 2 grams per day for the first week. You can do this by eating three large dill pickles, five large olives, or one chicken bouillon cube dissolved in water per day.

Dr. E. S. Garnett and colleagues performed a metabolic ward study in which seven obese females were placed on total-starvation diets (consuming only 115 milligrams of sodium per day). These authors found that while exchangeable sodium (the sodium that can move into and out of the extracellular fluid) fell during the first week of starvation, it progressively rose to prestarvation levels despite continued fasting and sodium restriction.[135] This occurred despite a large negative sodium balance, indicating that stored sodium (from either bone, skin, or organs) was being pulled into the exchangeable sodium space. These findings suggest that prolonged fasting on top of a low sodium intake pulls sodium from body stores (such as bone) to replenish the exchangeable sodium space. In essence, prolonged fasting, especially on top of a low sodium intake, may put patients at risk of osteoporosis, as sodium is an important component in bone formation and seems to be depleted while fasting.

We really cannot rely on blood sodium levels to know if someone is deficient in salt because the body maintains a normal blood sodium level at the expense of sodium depletion in other parts of the body. Despite starting with different levels of total body sodium, almost all patients stop losing sodium once they hit around 69 grams of total body sodium. In fact, 63 to 69 grams of total body sodium may indicate a *minimal* level of total body sodium required for humans to survive. Importantly, in one study, a patient who started with 151 grams of total body sodium lost 82 grams of sodium during total starvation, whereas the others patients lost much less. This study suggests that certain individuals function at a higher total body sodium content compared to others and, therefore, some are at less risk of salt deficit. That means some individuals are likely more susceptible to the harms of low-salt diets compared to others—and we need to determine just who those people are before we issue blanket recommendations about salt intake.[136]

You May Need More Salt to Prevent Iodine Deficiency

Iodization of salt has been an important public health victory for eliminating goiter around the world. In one study, 133 people were tested to see if salt restriction was related to iodine deficiency.[137] Half the subjects were placed on a normal-sodium diet and half were placed on a reduced-sodium-intake diet, and then twenty-four-hour sodium and iodide excretions were measured. The results indicated that those in the salt-restricted group consumed just 1.9 grams of sodium per day, and 50 percent of the patients excreted 100 micrograms or less of iodide per day at eight months. In other words, more than half of the subjects restricting their salt intake were probably not getting the daily recommended iodine intake—and these subjects were consuming *more* sodium than what is currently recommended by the American Heart Association (1.9 grams per day versus less than 1.5 grams per day, respectively) and meeting the WHO recommendations (less than 2 grams of sodium per day). However, only 25 percent of patients eating the normal-sodium diet excreted 100 micrograms or less of iodide per day at eight months. In essence, compared to people who do not restrict their salt intake, those who follow the low-salt advice may be twice as likely to not get the recommended daily amount of iodine.

In order to prevent goiter, one needs to consume 50 to 70 micrograms of iodine per day. Based on twenty-four-hour urinary iodide levels, 15 percent of people in the low-salt group were at risk of goiter compared to 10 percent of the control group—suggesting there's a 50 percent increased risk for developing goiter when on a low-salt diet (around 1.9 grams of sodium) versus a normal-salt diet. The risk is certainly higher in those who aren't eating foods naturally high in iodine. Importantly, approximately 50 percent of the individuals in this study ate seafood at least once a week, so this study may underestimate the risk of iodine deficiency in developing goiter for those who do not regularly eat the same amount of seafood. Interestingly, around the time of this study (1983–1984), iodophors were still being heavily used as cleaning agents in the dairy industry, which ensured that dairy products provided more iodine.[138] Thus, current populations, who consume dairy products without the same levels of iodophors, may be at even greater risk for iodine deficiency and goiters than the study group.

You May Need More Salt to Fight Infections

Our host-defense system may be driven by salt, which may activate other antimicrobial defense systems. Without salt, we wouldn't be able to effectively get rid of pathogens from the skin, as a hypertonic environment increases the production of nitric oxide, helping to eliminate pathogens.[139] This may be why salt excretion is substantially reduced in patients who have a fever and infection, in order to help combat the microbial invaders. Eating enough salt can ensure adequate salt deposits in our skin, which can help encourage protective macrophages to help attack bacterial infections. The authors of one study concluded, "Our findings suggest that edema formation in infection is not only characterized by water retention and swelling but also creates a microenvironment of high sodium concentration." The researchers found that in mice fed a high-salt diet, their "sodium reservoir" was particularly powerful in fighting off *L. major* bacterial infections, with salt serving an antimicrobial barrier function in the skin.

Eating a normal-salt diet may help us ward off skin infections. As we enter the days of antibiotic resistance, skin infections can potentially be lethal if they become systemic. Even scarier: low-salt diets may predispose us to a greater risk of complications, or even death, from methicillin-resistant *Staphylococcus aureus* (MRSA) and other skin infections or flesh-eating bacteria. MRSA is often treated with a medication called Bactrim/Septra (a combination of trimethoprim and sulfamethoxazole), which can cause kidney damage and metabolic acidosis that can also lead to salt wasting. Sulfamethoxazole causes increased sodium excretion by the kidneys, so patients receiving high doses of this medication may be at risk of sodium depletion.[140] Additionally, since salt is so important for fighting skin infection, a higher-salt diet may help diabetic patients heal their skin ulcers (a common complication). In essence, patients with diabetes may need even more salt to help prevent and treat skin ulcers. But the skin isn't the only organ that salt helps fight off infection. High concentrations of salt in lymphatic organs (lymph nodes, spleen, thymus) and inflamed tissue may help the body fight off infections.[141] A high-salt diet may also help in sepsis, as hypertonic saline increases T-cell function,[142] and may help in other systemic infections, such as human immunodeficiency virus (HIV) or other dangerous viruses such as Ebola or hepatitis.

Infections come via our food supply as well. Over one million cases of food poisoning in the United States happen every year (almost five hundred being fatal), and "low-salt" versions of packaged food products may have higher microbial counts than normal-salt versions, increasing the risk of food poisoning.[143] Hence, low-salt packaged foods may increase the risk of food-borne illness. Additionally, when you have food poisoning, you lose a lot of salt in your vomit and diarrhea.

Basically, low-salt diets may increase the risk of death in the over one million food poisoning cases just in the United States every year.

One study in Australia estimated that decreasing microbial growth rates by modest amounts can have a large effect on the risk of listeriosis from processed meats. The study authors said that "reducing the growth rate of L. monocytogenes by 50 percent decreased the risk of illness in the population by 80 to 90 percent."[144] This suggests that even a small increase in growth rate resulting from a decrease in salt without adequate adjustment of other preservative factors could considerably increase the risk to the susceptible population.

All of this indicates that lowering the salt content of food, in the effort to meet unscientific low-salt guidelines, may increase the risk of food-borne illness and the degree of food wastage. "One manufacturer producing reduced salt bacon has already used this technique; when the salt content of bacon was reduced from 3.5 percent to 2.3 percent, the shelf-life was reduced from 56 days to 28 days."[145] Lowering the salt content of packaged foods may also require higher use of suspect preservatives, such as phosphates, nitrates, and nitrites, in order to maintain microbial stability, which are likely more detrimental to our health compared to salt.[146]

YOU MAY ALSO NEED MORE SALT FOR . . .

- **Autism:** Autism is a complex disorder, with many likely causes and genetic links. However, one theory holds that autism could be a disorder of overhydration, with low sodium levels in the blood depleting certain essential brain nutrients, such as taurine and glutamine.[147] This may be one reason why children with autistic disorders tend to have salt cravings. Children with autism may benefit from consuming more salt, whereas low-salt diets may actually worsen their condition. Oral rehydration salts may also be of benefit in autism.[148]

- **Caffeine:** Caffeinated beverages, acting like natural diuretics, can increase water and salt loss from our kidneys. Coffee and tea are now the second and third most commonly consumed beverages around the world—not to mention other caffeinated drinks such as sodas and energy/sports drinks that flood the market. We are now more than ever a salt-excreting society, because of our caffeine addiction.

- **Certain conditions:** Hypotonic hyponatremia can be found in severe polydipsia (frequent among schizophrenic patients) or "beer drinker's hyponatremia" (also known as "beer potomania syndrome"—people who overconsume beer basically give themselves dilutional hyponatremia). Certain types of renal tubular acidosis and metabolic alkalosis cause hyponatremia, whereby the increased bicarbonate in the urine forces sodium to flow out of the kidneys.[149] Cerebral salt-wasting syndrome (from subarachnoid hemorrhage) can also cause low sodium levels in the blood. Euvolemic hyponatremia can be caused by hypothyroidism, primary adrenal insufficiency, and hypopituitarism with secondary adrenal insufficiency. Autoimmune Addison's disease (or other adrenal insufficiency disorders, such as adrenal fatigue) can also lead to hyponatremia.[150] Hyponatremia can also be caused by cortisol deficiency.[151]

- **Nicotine:** Those using forms of tobacco that contain nicotine (cigarettes, cigars, pipe and chewing tobacco) have an increased risk of low blood sodium levels due to nicotine's ability to increase water retention (via an increased production of antidiuretic hormone).[152]

Because of the many chronic disease states and medications that cause salt depletion in the Western world, we are now at a much greater risk of salt deficit than even primitive societies that eat very little salt. Thankfully, now that we recognize this, we can do something about it—and, in so doing, we can help ourselves prevent or even reverse many of today's most debilitating conditions. It's time for the Salt Fix. In the next chapter, I'll walk you through a step-by-step plan to help correct the salt balance in your body, reconnect with your innate salt thermostat, choose the best sources of high-quality salt for your situation, and help you drop the salt guilt, so you can get back to enjoying the vitality, energy, and delicious savory satisfaction that salt can bring.

The Salt Fix: Give Your Body
What It Really Needs

You've seen the evidence: your body needs more salt! Luckily, reversing your salt deficit is straightforward: simply by giving in to your innate, natural cravings, you can naturally guide yourself back to the ideal amount of salt your body needs to operate at its best. You've been taught to ignore those cravings and disregard your body's salt thermostat, so it can take a bit of time and experimentation to reset those internal protective mechanisms. Thankfully, just a few adjustments to your current diet and lifestyle can have significant, wide-ranging effects on your health.

I've created a five-step plan to help simplify the process of resetting your innate salt thermostat, reverse any current internal starvation, and bring your body back into its natural state of balance. I am laying these changes out in five steps so that they are manageable, with each step building on the one before. But you can follow these steps in a different order if that makes more sense to you in your life. You can even feel free to make all these changes right away! Do what feels best to you. But do try to incorporate some aspect of each of these steps, as doing so will ensure that you restore your body's preferred levels of life-giving salt.

There's no downside to this program. You'll enjoy more energy, fewer infections, improved sexual and athletic performance, and a faster metabolism. Your body will have increased immunity, better cellular function, and much less stress on critical organs. All you need to do is eat delicious foods with zero added calories! What could be better? Here's how to do it.

Step 1: Visit Your Doctor to Test for Internal Starvation

If you're storing fat around your middle or you're ravenously hungry all the time, and you have a low sodium intake *or* a high sugar intake, you may be worsening your underlying insulin resistance. And your elevated insulin levels could be nudging you closer toward or further into internal starvation. If these patterns sound familiar, consider scheduling a visit with your primary care physician.

Other signs that your insulin levels are out of whack and triggering internal starvation include the following:

- If you eat or drink something that's high in added sugars (generally more than 20 grams) and you become shaky, jittery, or sweaty afterward, that may mean that your body is oversecreting insulin and causing your blood sugar to crash.
- If you are diagnosed with nonalcoholic fatty liver disease, which affects approximately 30 percent of adults in the United States, that's another clue that you are probably suffering from internal starvation.

If this sounds like you, here's what to do:

Get your insulin levels checked. When you schedule your doctor's appointment, be sure to ask to have your fasting insulin level tested ahead of time. This will detect high insulin levels and indirectly let you know whether you're experiencing internal starvation, so you can discuss next steps during your doctor's visit.

Generally, a fasting insulin level of 5 uIU/mL or less is optimal; if it's higher than that, you'll probably store more fat than someone who has a lower fasting insulin level, even if both of you consume the same number and types of calories. To put this number in perspective, less-developed societies typically have a fasting insulin level of 3 to 5 uIU/mL; by contrast, in the United States the average fasting insulin is around 9 to 11 uIU/mL (though it has wavered a bit through the years).[1]

Seek out more nuanced testing. For more accurate results, you may consider requesting what's often called a "glucose challenge test" along with an insulin assay. In this test, your insulin and blood sugar levels are measured two hours after consuming a drink that contains 75 grams of glucose. The test helps to determine if you have a large blood sugar and insulin spike after a meal, often a better gauge of internal starvation. If you have a high fasting insulin or high postprandial (after a meal) insulin level, you probably have some degree of internal starvation, and those high insulin levels will cause you to store an abnormal amount of fat for each calorie consumed.

Reevaluate your medications. If the tests detect high insulin, you'll want to work with your physician to lower it. The first step is for your doctor to assess whether a medication you're taking could be causing insulin resistance/high insulin levels. Many common drugs—including the SSRI antidepressants, certain antipsychotic medications, diuretics and beta-blockers for hypertension, and more—may worsen insulin resistance. For each of these underlying health conditions, there may be other drugs or better options within the same class that can effectively treat what ails you without promoting high insulin levels. Depending on your fasting insulin and blood sugar levels, you may also want to discuss whether you'd benefit from taking an insulin-sensitizing medication (such as metformin, acarbose, or pioglitazone). The table on page 162 provides alternative medications that may help to prevent or reverse insulin resistance.

Consider These Medication Swaps to Prevent (or Reverse) Insulin Resistance

Current Medication	Suggested Alternative
Diuretics	
Hydrochlorothiazide	Indapamide
Beta-blockers	
Atenolol or Metoprolol	Carvedilol or Nebivolol
Statins	
Atorvastatin, Simvastatin, Rosuvastatin	Livalo® or Pravastatin
Anti-diabetic medications	
Glyburide, Glipizide, Glimeperide, Insulin, Repaglinide	Acarbose, Metformin, Pioglitazone
Angiotensin-converting enzyme (ACE) inhibitors	
Enalapril or Lisinopril	Perindopril

Step 2: Replace Simple Sugars with Real Salt

The adage about "moderation in all things" applies to the consumption of salt and sugar—but the definition of "moderation" may be *broader* than you thought it was for salt and much *narrower* than you believed it should be for sugar. Shoot for the sweet spot (so to speak):

- The *full* amount of salt you crave, enough to fulfill your body's needs and please your taste buds, without going overboard (no more than around 6,000 milligrams of sodium per day for someone who isn't wasting salt from their kidneys or not able to absorb salt well); and
- The *minimum* amount of sugar to satisfy your sweet tooth (striving to reduce whenever possible, and only on rare occasions eating more than 30 grams of added sugar, as more than that can compromise your health).

When patients come into the doctor's office with high blood pressure, the first recommendation that many doctors make is to reduce salt—but I believe so many lives could be saved if we urged patients to enjoy plentiful salt and cut way back on their sugar instead. Allowing yourself to eat as much salt as you crave can help you kick your sweet tooth.

For years, you've been told that in order to get your intake of salt in the right zone, you need to retrain your taste buds to live with less. But now you know your taste buds aren't what's driving your salt consumption—your internal salt thermostat *controls* your taste buds in order to raise or lower overall salt intake.

If you're ingesting more salt than normal—if you have a heavy hand with the saltshaker—your body is likely telling you that it needs that extra salt for optimal health. By contrast, the opposite is true of sugar; the sweet stuff can hijack your body and your brain, causing your intake of sugar to steadily increase to dangerous levels, all driven by cravings and dependence. Again, in contrast to salt, you *can* break that addiction by retraining your taste buds—and, as we discussed in chapter 6, increasing salt as you decrease sugar can help support your body to handle this transition in several other ways as well.

Some people find that an all-or-nothing approach to cutting sugar works well; others prefer a phased-in approach. I think it's a bit easier and more sustainable to gradually reduce your sugar, bit by bit, as you increase your salt. Regardless of which approach you choose, here are the optimal sugar guidelines to shoot for:

Go for 20 grams of sugar or less. Shoot to limit yourself to no more than 20 grams (about 5 teaspoons) per day of "added sugars" or "free sugars" (in fruit juices, syrups, and honey—this may not necessarily apply to raw wild honey, which contains a plethora of antioxidants). Note that this recommendation is independent of the natural sugars you might consume from fruits, vegetables, and other whole foods. In general, I recommend a 20/80 rule: consume no more than 20 grams of refined sugar per day, and follow this rule at least 80 percent of the time (eight out of ten days, for instance). If you can do this, you'll be well on your way to fixing a sugar addiction and improving your health.

Never drink your sugar. To cut sugar from your diet, the first place to start is by dropping any source of liquid-added or free sugars, such as soda, fruit juices (even 100 percent real fruit juice), smoothies, sweetened iced teas, energy drinks, sports drinks, and lattes/mocha drinks—even the teaspoons of sugar you add to your coffee. Liquid sugar is the worst because it's most rapidly absorbed and therefore leads to worse metabolic consequences than solid sources. The 40 grams of sugar you can drink in literally seconds from one can of soda floods you with a huge sugar load. All that sugar can override the body's ability to metabolize it, so cutting back on these sweet liquids (or, ideally, forgoing them entirely) helps you make the most impactful difference for your body in this one change. (Artificial sweeteners aren't the answer, either; read on for more about that.)

Root out hidden sugars. Once you've cut out the obvious sources of added sugar, start to avoid added sugars such as high-fructose corn syrup and sucrose in other processed foods. Research has found that simply reducing your intake of added fructose lowers chronically high levels of insulin and reduces insulin resistance—so this is an essential change to make.[2] Getting in the habit of reading food and ingredient labels on packaged foods can help reveal hidden sugars. Sugar goes by many different names—in addition to white granulated sugar, caster sugar, raw sugar, and brown sugar, there's evaporated cane juice, corn syrup, agave nectar, maple syrup, coconut palm sugar, and most things that end in *-ose* (maltose, dextrose, and so on).

Stay vigilant with "healthy" sugars. Some forms of sugar are touted as being "healthier" than others, and there actually is some truth to that, but it's truer to say that some sugars are more *harmful* than others. Physiologically speaking, fructose and glucose are metabolized differently in the body, so sugars that contain fructose are not the same as those that contain pure glucose. Despite their different flavors, textures, and colors, the nutritional value of most forms of sugar is quite comparable, though molasses contains trace amounts of calcium, iron, and potassium, and honey is highest in antioxidant and antibacterial properties. And while a given amount of any type of sugar has the same number of calories (16 per teaspoon), the calories from fructose are much more harmful.[3]

Agave syrup once bore a health halo because it has a low glycemic index—meaning it causes a milder rise in blood sugar when you consume it. But recently it's been vilified because it contains very large amounts of fructose, even more than high-fructose corn syrup (which has long been at the top of the do-not-fly list). The problem is that agave syrup and other sugars containing fructose can promote unhealthy inflammation and interfere with the appetite-regulating hormones (such as leptin and ghrelin), which can lead to weight gain, especially around the belly. Moreover, consuming lots of agave syrup likely increases your chances of developing insulin resistance, putting you at risk for diabetes or making diabetes harder to control if you already have it. Basically, when it's consumed, the fructose in agave syrup, sucrose (table sugar), or high-fructose corn syrup enters a cell like an out-of-control freight train, overwhelming the blood-sugar-regulation system, causing oxidative stress, inflammation, depletion of ATP (adenosine triphosphate, which supplies energy for numerous biochemical cellular processes), and insulin resistance. It's a harmful cascade of events, any way you slice it. Any combination of fructose and glucose can set this domino effect into motion. Learning the sixty or more names for different types of sugar is a step in the right direction and will help you avoid inadvertently consuming sugar. While sugar that solely contains glucose (such as dextrose or corn syrup) is not as bad for your health as other forms that contain both fructose and glucose (such as high-fructose corn syrup, sucrose, evaporated cane juice, brown sugar, and possibly even molasses), it still can lead to insulin resistance and unwanted weight gain.

Avoid fake sugars entirely. Most sugar substitutes aren't necessarily the answer. Basically, artificial sweeteners confuse your body: when sugar doesn't accompany the sweet taste of sugar substitutes, your appetite kicks into overdrive so that your body can get the sugar it thinks it deserves. This may cause you to seek out real sugar in your diet, and you may even end up consuming more of the sweet stuff. Additionally, any carbohydrate that comes along with diet drinks (burger bun, fries, etc.) may be absorbed more easily, spiking your glucose levels and leading to worse health outcomes.

Get your sweet tooth hooked on just barely ripe fruit. While you're rehabilitating your taste buds, if you start to crave a quick sugar fix, choose small amounts of sugar from solid forms—then eat it slowly and savor it! Eating a piece of just-barely-ripe fruit (some berries, a peach or nectarine, melon cubes, or even an apple or pear) may help. (Fully or overly ripe fruit has a higher sugar content because it lacks resistant starch.) Also, consuming sugar with protein can boost the satiety factor and diminish the rapid rise in blood sugar that would otherwise occur. A small portion of dark chocolate with almonds and sea salt should do the trick because the dark chocolate will provide the sweetness you crave, the sea salt will stimulate the release of the neurotransmitter dopamine (which controls the reward and pleasure centers in the brain), and the almonds offer long-lasting satiety. Having a good-quality organic chocolate protein shake (such as Svelte, which contains stevia instead of sugar) is also a good way to curb your sugar cravings healthfully while promoting satiety (thanks to the protein). Stevia is a natural plant compound that has been consumed for thousands of years as compared to chemically produced artificial sweeteners. Svelte helped me out when I would get a sudden urge for sugar. Just a few sips and my sweet tooth would dissipate, and after just a few months I didn't even need it anymore. Stevia, in small doses—at most 10 grams per day—may be used to help you wean yourself off a penchant for sweets.

Resist the "sugar" in savory carbs. Then cut way back on refined carbs such as white bread, white rice, white pasta, and even starchy vegetables such as white potatoes. (See "Guilt-Free Potatoes" on page 167 for the sole exception.) Other strategies include eating a healthy carbohydrate in small amounts, such as one slice of Ezekiel (sprouted grain) bread dipped in extra-virgin olive oil. This flourless bread provides the "sugar fix," and the olive oil provides additional

GUILT-FREE POTATOES

While traditional preparations of white potatoes can lead to tremendous surges in blood sugar, modifying their preparation slightly will allow you to keep these comfort foods on the table for special occasions. If you slightly undercook the potatoes and then allow them to cool for eight hours in the refrigerator prior to eating, the cooling process turns "starchy" potatoes into "fiber potatoes." You can purchase small potatoes (preferably organic) and prepare them by washing them and cutting them into quarters. Preheat the oven to 350°F. Place the quartered potatoes in a large bowl along with chopped onions and lightly drizzle with extra-virgin olive oil. Mix the potatoes and onions together and then place them in a glass baking pan. Sprinkle the potatoes and onions with salt and pepper and then throw them into the oven and bake for 40 to 45 minutes, until slightly undercooked. Cooking and then cooling potatoes increases their resistant starch levels, which lowers their glycemic index and helps encourage weight loss.

You can use this process with any potato, from white to sweet. And, of course, feel free to sprinkle your potato treat liberally with salt!

satiety as well as healthy phenolic compounds. One piece of Ezekiel bread contains only 14 grams of carbohydrates (3 grams of which are fiber, providing a net effective carb content of just 11 grams per piece). Moreover, Ezekiel bread seems to cause less of a blood sugar spike compared to other more refined breads, and it is also organic (so it doesn't contain artificial preservatives or vegetable oils). It also contains other types of healthy substances (such as barley, lentils, and organic sesame seeds, depending on which Ezekiel bread you buy—the sesame seed version is my favorite!). Keeping Ezekiel bread in the

SALT HELPS LOW-CARB EATERS THRIVE

If you're actively trying to lose weight, be extra careful to get enough servings of healthy salt. Remember, one of the most common weight-loss approaches—cutting carbs—causes you to become a salt waster, excreting more salt than you would on a more balanced diet during the first three to ten days, especially when you hit ketosis (near 50 grams of carbohydrates per day or less). When your insulin levels begin to drop, your body will excrete more salt, especially if you've had insulin resistance for a while—it's almost as if your kidneys need to be retrained to reabsorb sodium without the help of excess insulin. (You may have experienced this as what's sometimes referred to as "The Atkins Flu": low-carbohydrate diets like Atkins can cause a depletion of sodium and water, leading to dizziness, light-headedness, and low blood pressure.)

You want to increase your salt intake to match the additional salt loss by the kidneys and help prevent the subsequent rise in insulin levels to compensate for this. Most people need to drink more water and get an additional 2,000 milligrams of sodium per day—compared to their normal sodium intake—during the first week of carbohydrate restriction (again, around 50 grams of carbohydrates per day or less). Then, they should add an additional 1,000 milligrams of sodium per day during the second week to match increased salt losses. This extra sodium can easily be obtained from consuming 3 ounces of pickles, one chicken or beef bouillon cube (dissolved in warm water), five jumbo olives, 6 ounces of oysters, or 12 ounces of crabmeat.

CONSIDER SUGAR-TAMING SUPPLEMENTS

Additionally, if you are overweight, diabetic, or prediabetic, or you have fatty liver disease, you may get an extra "boost" from using certain supplements while you are trying to cut down on your intake of sugar.

- L-carnitine has been found to improve fatty liver, may help with weight/fat loss, and may help reduce hunger.[4] Supplementing with 1,000 milligrams of L-carnitine two to three times daily (taken on an empty stomach) for a few months may be helpful.

- Glycine, which is the smallest of the amino acids, has also been found to help mitigate some of the metabolic harms of sugar. Consuming 5 grams of glycine (preferably in powder form mixed with water) three times daily thirty to forty-five minutes prior to meals may help reduce high blood pressure, improve fatty liver disease, and drop a few extra pounds of fat.[5]

- Ensuring that you are consuming around 1,000 milligrams of EPA/DHA (the active ingredients in fish oil) will also increase your ability to burn fat and has been found to help with weight loss (particularly that stubborn fat around the belly and liver).

- If your dietary intake of iodine is not adequate (not eating foods high in iodine such as cranberries, seaweed [as in sushi wrappers], or yogurt), supplementing with iodine may be the next best choice. Purecaps (www .purecaps.com) hires a third-party company to regulate their supplements. This may be a good option, although only healthcare professionals are allowed to purchase and sell its products.[6]

refrigerator and then toasting it enhances its flavor, and dipping it in extra-virgin olive oil provides a great satiating healthy snack without causing the damage that a rapidly absorbed sugary snack would. Make sure to spice up the olive oil with some good garlic salt, spices, and perhaps a dash of pepper before dipping.

Note: if you have diabetes or prediabetes or are on any medication that may cause blood sugars to drop, make sure your doctor is aware that you plan on cutting back on consuming refined sugars and carbohydrates, especially if you take insulin. While there is debate if there is a true need (requirement) for dietary carbohydrates, this does not mean that there cannot be consequences when cutting your intake (like hypoglycemia, also known as low blood sugar), so make sure your doctor is in the loop.

Step 3: Focus on Whole, Salty Foods

One of the best things about doing the Salt Fix is getting a free pass to once again indulge in delicious, *real* high-salt foods. No need to sacrifice taste with the unsatisfying fake versions of your favorite foods. In fact, as you know by now, low-salt versions of processed foods may be detrimental to your health in the long run, possibly increasing your risk of food-borne illness, diabetes, obesity, metabolic syndrome, and hypertension. For example, store-bought pasta sauce is often loaded with sugar, and it doesn't need to be. When you follow the tenets of the Salt Fix, you can quickly prepare your own with tomato paste, diced tomatoes, herbs, minced garlic, salt to taste, and perhaps just a bit of added sugar, and your homemade version will be mouthwateringly tasty and have far less sugar than the one in the jar.

Also, don't forget that for most people your body constantly tells you to consume 3,000 to 5,000 milligrams of sodium per day, so if you avoid salt in your meals, this will likely cause you to consume more food throughout the day to get the amount of salt your body craves. Your body will eventually drive you to get more salt until you've hit that 3,000-to-5,000-milligrams-of-sodium mark—so if you consume low-salt versions of foods, you may end up eating two to three times as much because your body is still "hungry" for salt. Which may obviously mean more pounds in your near future, so try to avoid low-salt versions unless your body is telling you it has had enough.

Adding the right amount of salt to your meals can help you better control the composition of your plate. The correct salt can encourage you to increase your intake of fruits and veggies (especially the bitter ones) by making them taste better. When you gain more satisfaction from boosting the flavors of high-quality food, you'll eat more of what's good for you, and less of what's bad—which is what allows you to stop *overeating* refined foods that make you fat.

Emulate the world's most delicious cuisines. Many populations that eat a high-salt diet live long and in good health, such as those of France, Italy, South Korea, and Japan. The difference is that these cultures eat real unprocessed food and add salt, rather than consuming processed foods (that also just so happen to be high in salt). The Mediterranean diet, widely considered the most heart healthy, is not low in salt—think of the olives, sardines, anchovies, salted and cured meats, aged cheeses, soups, and so on! Go ahead and bring back those previously verboten high-salt foods. Dig into the nuts, pickles, sauerkraut, seafood, shellfish, beets, Swiss chard, seaweed, and artichokes—all are highly nutritious natural sources of sodium. (Bonus: many of these foods are also abundant in potassium, magnesium, and calcium, minerals that will help regulate your blood pressure.)

Seek out alternative iodine sources. To emulate these salt-rich cuisines, aim to eat whole foods that can help you get your iodine needs covered, such as dairy, eggs, seafood, sushi, seaweed, cranberries, and potatoes that have been undercooked and cooled (see page 167 for preparation information). Stick as close to nature as possible, such as fish from the ocean rather than farmed, and dairy/eggs from grass-fed and free-range sources.

Incorporate salts into every meal. For breakfast, start with some organic salted nuts—especially helpful if you drink coffee, to replace what is lost in the urine. For lunch, create your own homemade dressing with extra-virgin olive oil (preferably organic), organic garlic salt, pepper, and herbs—mix well and you have created a healthy dressing. Take this delicious salt-enhanced dressing and pour it over bitter greens or salads. You can even use this dressing as a dipping sauce for your meats. Other good options for lunch include organic salted cured meats with aged cheeses (preferably from free-range or pastured animals) with organic pickles or olives as a side. For dinner, if you're in the mood for some grass-fed meat, use olive oil to coat both sides, sprinkle liberal amounts of organic garlic salt on both sides with a dash of pepper, and sear each side over medium-high heat; then drop the temperature down to medium to avoid overcharring your meat.

Use salt to flavor label-free foods. Salt is the gateway to enhancing your food's flavor, allowing you to enjoy healthier bitter foods, to make healthy homemade dressings and sauces, and to just eat more *real* food. Real, whole foods—like fruits, vegetables, nuts and seeds, beans and legumes, and fish—don't need nutrition labels, so you can never really go wrong with eating foods that are label-free. Naturally occurring salts and fats can bring out the inherent flavors in whole foods and help make them more satisfying.

In particular, ocean fish that consume algae and have a high omega-3 fatty acid and salt content—such as salmon, mackerel, tuna, and sardines—will promote satiety and fat loss. If your hunger is in a state of overdrive due to internal starvation and high insulin levels, consuming healthy fats and lean proteins—in fatty fish, nuts, grass-fed beef, organic cheeses, olives, and the like—will help promote feelings of fullness and improve insulin sensitivity and leptin resistance.[7] And adding salt to healthy but generally less palatable foods (such as Brussels sprouts, cabbage, and turnips) will allow you to eat more of them.

Diversify flavors to wean yourself from sugar. Once you start consuming more real foods and fewer items with added sugars, your palate will grow accustomed to foods that are less sweet; you really *will* be retraining your taste buds, in the right direction this time! And before you know it, foods with even modest amounts of added sugar that used to taste good to you will taste too sweet—that's a very good thing! The key is to learn to consciously make healthy whole-food choices; pair ingredients smartly and use herbs and spices strategically. And when you're not craving salt but you need some extra flavor, add additional spices and herbs instead of sugar.

USING SALT IN THE BATTLE BETWEEN GOOD AND BAD BACTERIA

One theory that's been gaining traction in recent years is the notion that an imbalance between bad and good bacteria in the gastrointestinal system–your "gut microbiome"–may play a role in setting the stage for obesity. Simply put, consuming lots of sugar may promote the growth of harmful gut bacteria and *Candida albicans* (a type of yeast), microorganisms that can impede the absorption of nutrients by your cells, another form of internal starvation.[8]

By contrast, salt plays an essential role in promoting the growth of good bacteria in specific foods, which can foster health in the gut once you've consumed those foods. For example, using sea salt or brine to ferment foods like vegetables (say, in the preparation of kimchi or sauerkraut) helps preserve these foods naturally and create an environment where probiotics (the "good" bacteria) can flourish. These health-promoting bacteria are naturally present in foods such as yogurt and kefir but can also be created through the fermentation process. Research suggests that consuming probiotics regularly can lead to improved immune function, better digestive health, and possibly an enhanced ability to control your weight.

Step 4: Add in Naturally Higher-Nutrient Salt

Most kitchens have a shaker of unassuming white table salt close to the stove or table. We've grown so accustomed to this as our default salt that we can sometimes forget that salt doesn't just magically appear bleached white and perfectly granulated in nature! Not surprisingly, the healthier types of salts found in nature tend to be untouched by contaminants and less refined or processed. Salt naturally comes in many different flavors—smoky, earthy, nutty, peppery, sweet, or even sulfuric (smells like rotten eggs!). Experiment with different flavors to find your favorite. Some salts may have additional mineral content. Here's a look at the breakdown of some popular "natural" salts and how they compare with standard table salt.

Type of salt: **Redmond Real Salt**

Qualities: Sea salt with different texture varieties (coarse, granular, or powder); said to have a sweeter flavor than Himalayan salt

Nutrient profile: Provides sixty trace minerals and seems to have the highest calcium content of the popular sea salts. If your entire day's worth of salt (3,450 milligrams of sodium) came from Redmond Real Salt, you would get around 45 milligrams of calcium, 8 milligrams of magnesium, 9 grams of potassium, and 178 micrograms of iodine. If the company's own elemental analysis is correct, Redmond Real Salt may be a great way of helping you reach your recommended dietary allowance for iodine.

Purity issues: Apparently this salt does not contain anticaking agents, and it seems to lack the radioactive elements found in Himalayan salt. There also appears to be less subjection to environmental pollutants compared to salt obtained from modern oceans.[9]

Harvesting: Mined from an ancient seabed in Redmond, Utah.[10]

Type of salt: Celtic sea salt

Qualities: Light gray in color; coarse in texture; may be slightly damp (may require air-drying prior to placement into a saltshaker)

Nutrient profile: Provides eighty-two vital trace minerals but in rather low quantities. Celtic sea salt is touted for having the highest magnesium content of all the salts, but it may provide only around 40 milligrams of magnesium per day. Other trace minerals in an entire day's worth of Celtic sea salt include just 17 milligrams of calcium, 9 milligrams of potassium, and only 6 micrograms of iodine. To sum it up, the actual amount of almost all of these trace minerals (except perhaps the magnesium content) is so minimal that the added benefit may not be worth the added cost.[11]

Purity issues: This salt is supposedly not subjected to refinement or bleaching processes, and there are no additives in it; however, it is harvested from modern-day seas, which means it may contain traces of toxic metals such as mercury. However, it is said that Makai Pure Deep Sea Salt from the Selina Naturally Celtic Sea Salt collection is taken from the deep sea (2,000 feet below the ocean's surface). This part of the ocean supposedly does not mix with other parts of the ocean (because of the deep cold ocean currents) and hence that particular Celtic sea salt may possibly contain less contamination.[12]

Harvesting: Comes from a modern ocean and gets evaporated in ponds off the shores of France (hence, it is not subjected to very high heat as is regular table salt).[13]

Type of salt: Himalayan (pink) salt

Qualities: Pinkish in color; crystalized or chunky in texture; earthy flavor

Nutrient profile: Contains eighty-four minerals and trace elements and may have the most potassium of any of the sea salts (about three times as much potassium as Redmond Real Salt). To be fair, however, even if your total salt intake came from Himalayan salt, this would only provide around 28 to 32 milligrams of potassium (only a fraction of the daily recommended amount—4,700 milligrams).[14] To put this in perspective, 1 cup of black beans provides 2,877 milligrams of potassium. Himalayan salt is the most expensive of all the popular salt varieties.

Purity issues: It is generally mined by hand and hand-washed after being collected from unspoiled underground sources; hence, it is probably less contaminated by toxic metals but may have other radioactive elements such as radium, uranium, polonium, plutonium (although the concentrations are less than 0.001 part per million).[15]

Harvesting: Mined in different parts of Pakistan. Comes from an ancient dried-up ocean.[16]

Type of salt: **Himalayan black salt (kala namak)**

Qualities: Indian rock salt said to smell like rotten eggs because of its sulfur content. Brownish-pink to dark violet in color when whole, light purple to pink when ground.

Nutrient profile: Mainly consists of sodium chloride as well as sodium bisulfate, sodium bisulfite, sodium sulfide, iron sulfide, and hydrogen sulfide.

Purity issues: The purity depends on how it is produced. Kala namak is apparently widely used in Bangladesh, India, and Pakistan as a condiment.

Harvesting: It appears kala namak can be produced in numerous ways, either from natural halite (rock salt) of the Himalayan salt ranges (mined in Bangladesh, India, Nepal, and Pakistan) and the North Indian salt lakes (Sambhar Salt Lake or Didwana as well as the Mustang District of Nepal), or synthetically created by combining sodium chloride with sodium sulfate, sodium bisulfate, and ferric sulfate (apparently this is the most common way of production nowadays).[17]

Type of salt: Black and red Hawaiian sea salts*

Qualities: Hawaiian black lava salt is actually not a volcanic salt deep within the earth. It is made up of Pacific white sea salt crystals mixed with activated charcoal from burned-up coconut shells.[18] The activated charcoal supposedly provides antioxidants, has detoxifying properties, and may be good for digestion.[19] Hawaiian black lava salt is said to have a nutty or smoky flavor. Hawaiian red Alaea salt is also made up of white sea salt crystals, but it is infused with volcanic red clay (rich in iron oxides). Hawaiian red Alaea salt is said to have a sweet flavor.[20] These salts come as fine or coarse crystals that may be damp.

Nutrient profile: About 94 percent consists of sodium chloride. An entire day's worth of Hawaiian sea salt may provide 30 to 35 milligrams of magnesium, 18 milligrams of potassium, 11 to 14 milligrams of calcium, and little to no iodine. Black Hawaiian sea salt seems to contain the highest amount of iron of all the naturally occurring salts (up to 3 milligrams of iron in a full day's worth of salt).

Purity issues: The Pacific Ocean near Hawaii may be less contaminated than other parts of the ocean. The Hawaii Kai Corporation website provides the authentic Hawaiian salt from Molokai (supposedly the most isolated island, and because of this the salt here may have the least contamination from pollution). The sea salt harvested by the Hawaii Kai

* Also known as Hawaiian black lava salt and Hawaiian red Alaea salt. However, pink, green, white, and gray Hawaiian sea salts are also available, but they are not as popular or as traditional to the islands as the black and red salts.[21]

Corporation is "apparently under the supervision of certified salt masters, who are members of the Salt Masters Guild of Hawaii, an association formed with the goal of reinvigorating the thousand-year tradition of salt making as practiced by the ancient Hawaiian culture."[22] However, you can get other good Hawaiian salts from the other islands.[23] Beware of imitation salts that are "produced by mechanically mixing a cheap, highly refined California sea salt (about 99.8 percent pure sodium chloride) with alaea clay from China or Hawaii. Typically the darker the red color, the higher the quality of alaea clay used to make it."[24]

Harvesting: Solar-evaporated Pacific sea salt.[25]

Type of salt: Table salt (aka sodium chloride)

Qualities: Fine white crystals

Nutrient profile: Contains only two minerals—sodium and chloride—because the rest have been stripped away; if it's iodized, however, it will also contain iodine, which was added to table salt in the 1920s to prevent iodine-deficiency goiter (an abnormal enlargement of the thyroid gland).

Purity issues: It is usually highly refined and heavily ground, and most of the impurities have been removed. The trouble is, finely ground salt tends to clump together, so various additives, called anticaking agents, are added to ensure that it flows freely; the safety of some of these agents is questionable, but so far there does not seem to be much of a concern.

Harvesting: Mined throughout various parts of the world.[26]

Nutrient Comparison of the Most Popular Salts

This table contains estimated mineral contents (which will vary from product to product) and is based on an entire day's worth of salt intake from each salt.

	Iodized Table Salt	Redmond Real Salt	Celtic Sea Salt	Hawaiian Sea Salts	Himalayan (Pink) Salt
Iodine	450 mcg*	178 mcg	6mcg	Little to none	<100–250mcg
Calcium	0 mg	45 mg*	17 mg	11–14 mg	37 mg
Magnesium	0 mg	8 mg	40 mg*	30–35mg	1.4 mg
Potassium	0 mg	9 mg	9 mg	18 mg	28–32 mg*

*Indicates the salt with the highest content of that mineral.

As discussed earlier, the actual amounts of additional trace minerals provided by the sea salts are fairly minimal, except for the iodine (and perhaps calcium) contained in Redmond Real Salt and perhaps the magnesium content in Celtic sea salt and Hawaiian sea salts. If you are not obtaining an adequate intake of iodine, using Redmond Real Salt may provide some advantages. If your diet lacks calcium or magnesium, Redmond Real Salt and Celtic Sea Salt, respectively, may provide some additional health benefits compared to plain table salt. However, eating real foods will provide at least ten times the amount of these trace minerals.

Perhaps the most significant difference between table salt and the popular sea salts listed here is in the processing. Table salt is said to be bleached (to make it pure white) and treated with high heat (around 1,200°F) and anticaking agents (so the salt doesn't clump together).[27] However, the sea salts seem to lack this type of processing, which may provide a higher level of reassurance regarding their safety.

The best salt (in my opinion) would be Redmond Real Salt for five main reasons:

1. It seems to be the cheapest of the popular sea salts.
2. It provides a meaningful amount of iodine.
3. It may have the least contamination (as it comes from an

ancient dead sea, whereas Celtic sea salt, for example, comes
from a modern ocean).

4. It seems to have fewer radioactive elements compared to
   Himalayan salt.

5. It does not come as damp crystals (unlike sea salts from
   modern oceans) and thus does not require any air-drying.

If you are unlikely to obtain the recommended daily amount of
iodine (150 micrograms per day for most people) from your diet, either Redmond Real Salt or iodized table salt may be a good choice for
you. Otherwise, you may want to supplement with additional iodine.

Vegans are particularly at risk of iodine deficiency, as some of the
most common food sources containing substantial amounts of iodine
include dairy, eggs, shellfish/seafood, and sushi (vegans can obtain
iodine from seaweed, cranberries, and baked potatoes). For example,
it is estimated that one sushi roll contains around 92 micrograms of
iodine, mostly from the seaweed (according to Food Standards Australia New Zealand).[28]

My recommendation would be to first try to obtain iodine from
your diet. Since rigorous studies have yet to be performed, you should
probably not solely rely on iodine-containing salt to obtain your daily
iodine intake. The main purpose for eating salt is for obtaining sodium and chloride. If your diet is not adequate in iodine (or you are
losing good quantities of iodine from sweat) and you do not want to
use iodine supplements, then consuming Redmond Real Salt or iodized table salt may be a good option for you.

If iodine intake is not a concern, then using any organic salt or
organic garlic salt is also a good option, as it may save you money
compared to the popular sea salts and should be less processed compared with table salt. The real benefit of these less-processed salts may
come from the reduced environmental contamination and processing, although this is certainly debatable. The additional cost of these
more expensive sea salts ranges from three to ten times the cost of
regular table salt.

ACCEPT NO SALT SUBSTITUTES

Sometimes people who are avoiding salt on recommendations from their doctor turn to salt substitutes. But they aren't necessarily the answer, either. For one thing, many salt substitutes contain potassium and chloride (such as AlsoSalt)[29] instead of sodium chloride, and people with kidney problems often have trouble processing potassium chloride or getting rid of the excess. If you have chronic kidney disease or you take certain antihypertensive medications (such as ACE inhibitors or potassium-sparing diuretics), the extra buildup of potassium could lead to potassium overload (a condition called hyperkalemia), which can be fatal if it's not treated promptly. Go for the healthiest option: real salt!

Step 5: Let Salt Fuel Your Exercise

If you've found yourself short on energy and enthusiasm for exercise, once you start to address these core dietary issues, you may find yourself newly energized and motivated to hit the gym.

If you've been sedentary for a time, a good starting point is to increase your level of physical activity (under your doctor's supervision) with modest moderate forms of exercise such as going for a twenty-minute brisk walk or bike ride. But please don't stop there—also implement weight training, because lifting weights or doing resistance exercises (using resistance bands, weight machines, or your own body weight) is one of the best ways to help with insulin resistance. While aerobic exercise helps your body use insulin better and decreases storage of visceral (abdominal) fat, resistance training makes your body more sensitive to insulin and helps your muscles take up more glucose (sugar) from the blood, thereby lowering blood sugar. Even simply exercising before or right after you eat something with higher carbohydrate levels can help reduce any resulting swings in your blood sugar and insulin release.

Start slow and low, and build from there. Begin with walking and slowly increase to jogging and then running; start with light weights, and slowly increase to heavier weight lifting. In one 2012 study, researchers from the University of Verona in Italy found that after forty people with type 2 diabetes did aerobic training or resistance training for four months, both groups improved their insulin sensitivity and reduced their abdominal fat.[30] Meanwhile, a 2012 study from the Norwegian University of Science and Technology in Trondheim found that both maximal resistance training and endurance resistance training led to decreased insulin resistance in people who were at risk for developing type 2 diabetes. Interestingly, the maximal approach, which uses heavy loads to increase muscle power and force, led to a greater increase in the muscles' capacity for taking up glucose (sugar) from the blood, whereas the endurance type of resistance training brought greater insulin sensitivity.[31] One way or another, with increased exercise, your body will become better at soaking up sugar from your blood, and the carbohydrates you do eat will be less damaging as a result.

Of course, the more you exercise, the more salt your body will need, as you'll be losing salt through your sweat. Importantly, eating the appropriate amount of salt will help you retain the appropriate amount of water, so you'll be more hydrated and thus have more energy to exercise in the first place. Just 1 teaspoon of salt improves your stamina; it gives you a much more intense "pump" due to an increase in blood circulation, blood volume in the arteries is increased as water is pulled into the arteries, and your organs are perfused better. By avoiding salt, avid exercisers limit themselves, increasing side effects and dangerous risks of "circulatory collapse," and decreasing gains at the gym. I tell this to all my athlete friends: salt is the gateway to stronger muscles, longer stamina, and an increasingly sculpted physique.

Even if you're not at peak fitness level yet, eating enough salt is a great way to increase your energy levels, which will help you *want*

SALT SAVED MY EXERCISE PROGRAM

I relearned this lesson the hard way. A few years ago, it had been eight months since I was at the gym. (I had stopped at the end of the summer and only lifted light weights at home during the long eight-month winter.) My first day back, I asked the woman at the desk if I could sign up for another year and she told me to do my workout and check back in after I was done. After about an hour of lifting weights, I was heading back to the desk when I felt extremely light-headed and the room felt like it was spinning. I told the woman that I had to sit down for a second but I didn't want to let her know how bad I actually felt.

Well, there was no hiding it—I immediately collapsed onto a weight bench headfirst because my body was so exhausted. I went completely limp, facedown, closing my eyes, with only the ability to take deep breaths. I felt like a hundred-pound weight was on top of me, making me immobile. I felt like a fish out of water, neck turned to the side, taking gulps of air while lying prostrate. It was the most helpless I've ever felt.

After about three minutes of complete exhaustion and inability to move, I got enough strength to walk back over to the desk, and that was when I remembered: I had forgotten to take salt prior to my workout!

The next day before I went to the gym, I swallowed a full teaspoon of dry garlic salt and washed it down with water. I immediately felt invigorated. At the gym, not only was I able to lift heavier, longer, and with more intensity, but I sprinted for a mile after my workout without feeling any exhaustion. Contrast this with the day before, when I ended my workout not with a run but with near unconsciousness!

to exercise, one of the best things you can do for improving internal starvation. Best of all, when you stop restricting your salt intake, your insulin levels can start to drop toward the normal range, and your body will start to access its stored energy—in other words, you'll burn more fat! Your body will also use the calories you consume from food for energy, rather than immediately hoarding those calories as fat. More importantly, your salt-retaining hormones will go down, improving the sensitivity of your fat cells to insulin. Because of this, your fat cells can begin to absorb any extra fat and glucose—exactly where it's supposed to go, rather than being driven into your belly and internal organs. Your brain will become more sensitive to leptin, your natural appetite controls will return, and you'll have enough energy to exercise and feel good. Ultimately, by rebooting your internal salt thermostat—and achieving your long-lost normal salt intake—you'll help restore your vim and vigor, avoid reentering a state of internal starvation, turn up your slogging metabolism, and regain control of your weight. You will finally shift away from being "thin on the outside and fat on the inside" and move toward being "thin on the outside as well as the inside"! And best of all, you'll be able to kick that toxic sugar habit, once and for all.

All of these benefits flow directly from honoring your innate salt cravings; enjoying healthful, real food again; and allowing your body to eat the salt it so desperately wants and needs—instead of depriving yourself of one of your body's most elemental needs.

After you've completed this program, you'll be looking forward to a lifetime of eating good, tasty, healthy foods that support your health. You'll be free of endless hunger and destructive sugar cravings. You'll learn to listen to your salt thermostat; you'll dose yourself appropriately for peak performance and pay attention to the salt wasters that can creep into your lifestyle, such as caffeine and heavy sweating and medications. Over time, you'll develop an intuitive sense for when you need an extra shake of salt. You'll be living in tune with your body.

Not bad for a little dash of salt, huh?

Reach for the Right White Crystal

After reading this book, hopefully you're wise to the dietary deception that's been perpetrated on us all, and you have a sense of the tremendous effect the Salt Wars have had on our bodies and our health for over four decades. Rather than denying yourself the pleasures of this essential mineral, now is the time to welcome salt back to the table and embrace it as something that could help your body feel and function better. We need to move past the outdated, disproven salt–blood pressure hypothesis and consider what salt has done for us throughout human evolution. We need to remember:

Salt makes food taste great. By consuming more salt you can eat more healthy foods, which are often bitter and greatly improved by salt. Salt is our gateway to eating healthy. When you consume healthy foods that are high in magnesium, calcium, and potassium, salt should not increase blood pressure.

Salt restriction may lower blood pressure—but this isn't a good thing! A reduction in blood pressure with salt restriction isn't necessarily healthy. It generally indicates problems with low blood volume or dehydration. So while your blood pressure may be lower, your circulation is down, your organs are working harder, and the oxygen and nutrient supply to your organs is down—the opposite of long-term health the guidelines profess to protect.

Salt restriction raises heart rate. Any dehydration-related blood pressure reduction you may get from salt restriction is going to be off-set by the larger increase in heart rate. So while you may see a 2 percent reduction in your blood pressure, most people have a 10 percent increase in heart rate. This increase in heart rate is probably more harmful than the small drop in blood pressure, increasing the amount of stress on your heart and arteries, potentially leading to hypertension, heart failure, and cardiovascular events.

Salt restriction increases levels of harmful hormones. Restricting the intake of salt increases the levels of hormones that are known to enlarge and stiffen the heart and arteries. In other words, eating more salt may prevent the development of hypertension and heart failure, whereas restricting salt may actually *cause* these diseases! Low-salt diets also increase your risk of obesity by increasing insulin levels. Put plainly: eating more salt may keep us thin.

Salt may be one solution to—rather than a cause of—our nation's chronic disease crises. We've seen that a low salt intake could be promoting weight gain, high blood pressure, type 2 diabetes, kidney problems, heart attacks and strokes, thyroid disorders, falls and injuries, and possibly even premature death. It's important to remember that the same risks come when living in any salt-depleted state, whether it's because you've been dutifully following the low-salt guidelines, or you're athletic, or you have an underlying health condition or take a medication that depletes salt from your body. We need to start thinking carefully and critically about the level of *salt in our bodies* rather than trying to police *our salt intake*. Indeed, instead of putting out guidelines limiting the amount of salt in processed foods, the FDA should forgo limiting salt altogether. Doing so will prevent food manufacturers from being forced to substitute other, more potentially dangerous substances, such as artificial preservatives or sugar, in their place. Until the FDA gets the memo, here are a few ways we can all fight back against the low-salt propaganda.

WHAT CAN YOU DO?

❑   Start eating real food and salting to taste.

❑   Talk to your friends and family about the ideas in this book.

❑   Discuss the ideas in this book with your medical caregivers.

❑   Stop eating refined sugar, which is the true hypertension culprit.

WHAT CAN DOCTORS DO?

❑   Stop telling your patients that they should consciously restrict their salt intake; their bodies know better than any guidelines when it comes to salt intake.

❑   Educate yourself on the contraindications of the low-salt guidelines, and discuss these conflicts with your colleagues and hospital or practice administrators.

❑   Become a vocal advocate for removing low-salt recommendations among your peers in the medical community.

WHAT CAN POLICY MAKERS DO?

❑   Discuss the ideas in this book with colleagues and experts. Challenge those who rest on "received knowledge" to back up their assumptions with evidence and high-quality studies.

❑   Join the growing chorus of voices urging the FDA to remove its voluntary sodium reduction policy aimed at food manufacturers.

❑   Petition New York City lawmakers to remove warnings about "high-salt" foods in restaurants, ballparks, and movie theaters (i.e., a saltshaker outlined in an ominous black triangle).

Meanwhile, we should all focus on limiting our intake of the more harmful white crystal—sugar—for the sake of our waistlines, our health, and our longevity. Even if consuming lots of sugar doesn't lead to obesity for you, your sweet tooth could be silently and stealthily killing you by triggering chronic inflammation in your body, wreaking havoc with your hormones, causing oxidative stress, and triggering other forms of coronary or inflammatory damage that can increase your risk of having a heart attack or stroke, developing high blood pressure or type 2 diabetes, or getting Alzheimer's disease, fatty liver disease, or certain forms of cancer. *Nothing good ever comes from consuming loads of sugar.*

And yet it's hard to resist—and food manufacturers know this. Their goal is to engineer processed, packaged foods that are inherently irresistible so that you keep coming back for more—so they routinely, consciously, and deliberately add addictive sugar to their products. Government policies need to stop subsidizing bad foods and start supporting healthy foods. Encourage and support proposals to tax sugary foods, such as the soda taxes implemented in Berkeley, California, and Mexico, which are great examples of how taxing sugary beverages leads to a reduction in their intake. Slapping graphic warning labels on junk foods would also be a move in the right direction. Imagine seeing a diabetic ulcer on a soda can, a fatty liver next to a normal liver on a package of cookies, or a six-month-old infant who has become obese from drinking sugary baby formula on the label. You'd be much less likely to buy that product, wouldn't you?

Until those built-in disincentives become a reality, there are many different ways you can kick the sugar habit on your own, as you've seen in this book. One of the most powerful and impactful is to simply eat more salt. Cheap, delicious, versatile, lifesaving: salt is a powerful ally in our fight for a clean, healthful food supply. Remember: you could live the rest of your life without eating another granule of sugar, but you can't stay alive for very long without salt.

Hopefully, the tide is turning and our public health policy makers recognize this. We need to cut out the sugar and start celebrating salt. I call on all of us—individuals, parents, physicians, policy makers—to worry less about salt and pay way more attention to sugar, the *truly* toxic white crystal. Our very future depends on it.

In the meantime, please enjoy, guilt-free, one of nature's oldest and most pleasurable health safeguards, at every meal. Break out the saltshaker—for your taste buds and your health!

APPENDIX 1

. . . .

100-YEAR TIME LINE COVERING THE IMPORTANT HISTORICAL EVENTS RELATING TO SALT AND SUGAR

1904 and 1905—Ambard and Beauchard are given credit for launching the salt–blood pressure hypothesis and the belief that hypertension is caused by a retention of salt.[1]

1907—Lowenstein did not confirm the benefit of a low-salt diet for hypertension.[2]

1920s—Beginning of the Salt Wars in the United States.[3]

1920/1922—Allen, Scherrill, and coworkers promote the idea that salt increases blood pressure in those with and without kidney disease.[4]

1929—Berger and Fineberg conclude that low-salt diets (less than 1 gram of salt per day) are ineffective for treating hypertension in almost three out of four patients with essential hypertension.[5]

1930–1944—Low-salt diets slowly fall out of favor for the treatment of hypertension.[6]

1944–1948—Kempner shows benefit of his Rice Diet (which was, among other things, low in salt).[7]

1945—Grollman is credited for confirming that it was the low-salt part of Kempner's Rice Diet that lowered blood pressure.[8] However, the study actually showed that not all patients benefited, others experienced harm (one patient actually died), and another patient experienced circulatory collapse (which was fixed by providing salt to the patient).[9]

1950s—Lewis Dahl and George Meneely begin to suggest that salt is important in hypertension and chronic disease.[10]

1950s—The beginning of a debate, largely between the ideas of Ancel Keys and John Yudkin, regarding saturated fat versus sugar as a cause of heart disease.[11]

1960—Lewis Dahl publishes a famous paper correlating higher sodium intake with a higher prevalence of hypertension in only five populations.[12] This graph is very similar to the evidence Ancel Keys used to demonize dietary fat as a cause of coronary heart disease back in 1953.[13]

1961—Keys's "diet-heart hypothesis" is accepted by the American Heart Association. The idea of too much saturated fat, not sugar, is embraced as the dietary culprit causing heart disease.[14] Consequentially, the AHA recommends restriction of animal fats and an increase in the intake of vegetable oils to reduce the risk of heart disease.

1966—Hall and Hall show that sugar has a hypertensive effect in rats.[15]

1972—The *New England Journal of Medicine* publishes a paper by John Laragh and colleagues, which states, "Plasma renin activity emerges as a potential risk factor for patients with essential hypertension." Additionally, the study showed that a lower sodium intake correlated with higher plasma renin activity.[16]

1974—Richard A. Ahrens publishes a review paper suggesting that sugar is a driver of hypertension and heart disease.[17]

1974—The Food and Nutrition Board indicates that there is little direct evidence that hypertension is produced in people with normal blood pressure on a normal-sodium diet.[18]

1975—Alexander Walker writes that there is no definitive data that a high-sugar diet is a driver of heart disease or hypertension. His research seemed to have partial grants from the sugar industry.[19]

1976—Edward Freis and Meneely and Battarbee publish influential review papers on the harms of salt.[20]

1977—The Dietary Goals recommend that all Americans restrict their salt intake to 3 grams per day.[21]

1978—A. E. Harper publishes a critique of the 1977 Dietary Goals showing that the evidence for low-salt diets in hypertensive patients was inappropriately extrapolated to the general public and that a 3-gram daily salt intake was unrealistic and unattainable.[22]

1979—F. Olaf Simpson publishes a review paper that is skeptical of the benefits derived from a low-salt diet.[23]

1980—J. D. Swales publishes a review paper concluding that it was premature to recommend population-wide sodium reduction.[24]

1980—Preuss and Preuss show that sugar (without a high salt intake) increases blood pressure in rats with normal kidney function.[25]

1981—Yamori shows that as long as the Na/K ratio is less than 6 (despite a high sodium intake) in the Japanese, then the mean blood pressure is not hypertensive.[26]

1982—*Time* magazine releases its issue titled "Salt: A New Villain?"[27]

1983—Tessio Rebello and colleagues may have been the first to show that sugar significantly raises blood pressure in humans.[28] This was after we had vilified salt as the main dietary culprit causing hypertension.

1983—Robert E. Hodges and Tessio Rebello publish a review paper showing that sugar increases blood pressure in both animals and humans.[29]

1985—Boon and Aronson's review paper concludes that the amount of salt that needs to be restricted to obtain a measurable effect on blood pressure was intolerable for most patients.[30]

1988—Intersalt shows that when the four primitive societies were removed (leaving a total of forty-eight populations), a higher sodium intake did not correlate with a higher median blood pressure or prevalence of hypertension. Importantly, "body mass index had strong, significant independent relations with blood pressure in individual subjects."[31]

1989—Harriet P. Dustan states that there is no relation between blood pressure and salt depletion/salt loading, and that "salt-dependent hypertension" is not strictly controlled by salt intake but rather is probably controlled by aldosterone, norepinephrine, and epinephrine.[32]

1991—The first meta-analysis (which included nonrandomized and randomized trials) looking at sodium restriction and blood pressure is published.[33] Based only on reductions in blood pressure, the authors concluded, "Salt reduction by 100 mmol/24h would reduce mortality from ischaemic heart disease by an estimated 30 percent in the long term," and "A 50 mmol/24 h reduction in sodium intake would reduce the incidence of stroke by a fifth and that of ischaemic heart disease by a sixth."

1993—The Fifth Report of the Joint National Committee on Prevention, Detection, Evaluation, and Treatment of High Blood Pressure (JNC 5) cites the recently published 1991 meta-analysis to support sodium reduction.[34]

1995—Michael Alderman and colleagues publish a paper showing that "low urinary sodium is associated with greater risk of myocardial infarction among treated hypertensive men."[35]

1998—Niels Graudal publishes a meta-analysis of strictly randomized trials testing a low-sodium diet. The results found minimal reductions in blood pressure, whereas low-density lipoprotein (LDL) cholesterol, total cholesterol, noradrenaline, renin, and aldosterone were increased with a low-sodium diet. Their conclusion was, "These results do not support a general recommendation to reduce sodium intake."[36]

2001—The DASH-Sodium trial is published. This is a thirty-day randomized study that shows that reducing sodium intake may provide blood-pressure-lowering benefits.[37] However, it provided little benefit in those who had normal blood pressure and in those without hypertension who were forty-five years old and younger.[38] Additionally, there were increases in triglycerides, low-density lipoprotein (LDL), and total-cholesterol-to-high-density-lipoprotein (TC:HDL) ratio in those on the control diet when they restricted their salt intake.[39]

2002—Raben and colleagues show that a diet high in sugar significantly increases blood pressure in humans.[40]

2008—Brown and colleagues show that sugar raises blood pressure, heart rate, and cardiac output in humans, and that sugar increases blood pressure variability and myocardial oxygen demand.[41] These authors also show that sugar's antihypertensive effect occurs after its ingestion.

2010—Perez-Pozo and colleagues show that a high-sugar diet significantly increases twenty-four-hour ambulatory blood pressure in just a few weeks.[42]

2011—Stolarz-Skrzypek and colleagues publish a prospective population study concluding, "Lower sodium excretion was associated with higher cardiovascular disease mortality."[43]

2014—Malik and colleagues publish a systematic review of twelve studies (cross-sectional and prospective cohort) encompassing over 400,000 participants, showing that sugar-sweetened beverage intake is significantly associated with higher blood pressure and an increased incidence of hypertension.[44]

2014—Te Morenga and colleagues publish a meta-analysis of randomized controlled trials showing that a high-sugar diet significantly increases blood pressure versus a lower-sugar diet (the effect is around twice that found with altering sodium intake).[45]

2014—Adler and colleagues publish the most up-to-date Cochrane meta-analysis of randomized controlled trials indicating minimal reductions in blood pressure with a low-sodium diet and no significant reductions in all-cause mortality or mortality due to cardiovascular disease.[46]

2014—Graudal and colleagues publish a meta-analysis of twenty-three cohort studies and two follow-up studies of randomized controlled trials in 274,683 patients concluding that "compared with usual sodium intake, low- and excessive-sodium diets are associated with increased mortality."[47]

2015—Dietary Guidelines for Americans removed the severe limit on sodium intake (i.e., 1,500 milligrams per day), but the 2,300-milligram sodium limit remains.[48]

2016—Low sodium intakes are associated with an increased risk of cardiovascular events and death in those with or without hypertension, whereas high sodium intakes are associated with these harms only in hypertensive patients from a pooled analysis of four studies.[49]

2016—Patients without hypertension have no significant reduction in blood pressure with sodium restriction based on a meta-analysis of clinical studies.[50]

1977—*1st Edition of the Dietary Goals:* set an upper intake of sodium at 1.2 grams (3 grams of salt).[51]

1977—*2nd Edition of the Dietary Goals:* set an upper intake of sodium at 2 grams (**5 grams of salt**).[52]

1980—*Dietary Guidelines for Americans:* "**use less table salt**," avoid "pickled foods, salted nuts," "do not add salt to baby food," we "eat much more sodium than we need," and "the major hazard of excessive sodium is for *persons who have high blood pressure.*"[53]

1985—*Dietary Guidelines for Americans:* "**avoid too much sodium.**"[54]

1990—*Dietary Guidelines for Americans:* "**use salt or sodium only in moderation.**"[55]

1995—*Dietary Guidelines for Americans:* **Daily Value for sodium is 2,400 milligrams per day (6 grams of salt).**[56]

2000—*Dietary Guidelines for Americans:* "**Healthy children and adults need to consume** only small amounts of salt to meet their sodium needs—**less than ¼ teaspoon of salt daily.**"[57]

2005—*Institute of Medicine (IOM):* introduces an **adequate intake** (AI) of 1,500 milligrams and **upper level** (UL) of intake of 2,300 milligrams for sodium.[58]

2005—*Dietary Guidelines for Americans:* All Americans should consume less than 2,300 milligrams of sodium (about 1 teaspoon of salt) per day[59] (based on the IOM report). "*Individuals with hypertension, blacks, and middle-aged and older adults. Aim to consume no more than 1,500 mg of sodium per day.*"

2010—*Dietary Guidelines for Americans:* "*Reduce daily sodium intake to less than 2,300 mg and further reduce intake to 1,500 mg among persons who are 51 and older and those of any age who are African American or have hypertension, diabetes, or chronic kidney disease.*"[60]

2015—*Dietary Guidelines for Americans:* remove the severe sodium restriction recommendation (i.e., 1,500 mg of sodium per day) but keep the recommendation that all Americans should restrict their sodium intake to less than 2,300 mg per day.[61]

TIME LINE COVERING THE RECOMMENDATIONS FOR SUGAR INTAKE

1977—*Dietary Goals 1st edition:* **15 percent added sugars**[62]

1977—*Dietary Goals 2nd edition:* **10 percent refined and processed sugars**[63]

1980—*Dietary Guidelines for Americans:* "*Contrary to widespread opinion, too much sugar in your diet does not seem to cause diabetes.*" And "**avoid excessive sugars.**"[64]

1985—*Dietary Guidelines for Americans:* "**Avoid too much sugar**" and "*contrary to widespread belief, too much sugar in your diet does not cause diabetes.*"[65]

1990—*Dietary Guidelines for Americans:* "**Use sugar only in moderation**" and "Diets high in *sugar have not been shown* to cause diabetes."[66]

1995—*Dietary Guidelines for Americans:* "**Choose a diet moderate in sugars.**" It's as if the guidelines want us to eat added sugar.[67]

2000—*Dietary Guidelines for Americans:* "**Choose beverages and foods to moderate your intake of sugars.**" This is the first time that the Dietary Guidelines no longer state that "sugar doesn't cause diabetes" or that "there's no proof sugar causes diabetes."[68]

2002—*Institute of Medicine (IOM):* allows for 25 percent of total calories to come from added sugars.[69]

2005—*Dietary Guidelines for Americans:* 267 calories of "discretionary" calories (coming from added sugars and/or solid fat) are allowed; this would be only **67 grams of added sugars** (267/4 calories per gram of sugar = 67). However, it states that **up to 72 grams of added sugars are allowed.**[70] ("If fat is decreased to 22 percent of calories, then 18 teaspoons [72 g] of added sugars is allowed.")

2010—*Dietary Guidelines for Americans:* **technically up to 19 percent of total calories can be ingested from added sugars** if someone consumes 3,000 calories per day (the guidelines don't specifically state this, but if no solid fats are ingested, then 19 percent of calories from added sugars may be consumed).[71]

2015—*Dietary Guidelines for Americans:* finally recommends that added sugars should make up no more than 10 percent of total calories.[72]

APPENDIX 2

. . . .

DRUGS THAT CAN INCREASE NEED FOR SALT

Hypovolemic hyponatremia can be caused by thiazide and loop diuretics, sodium-glucose cotransporter 2 (SGLT2) inhibitors (like dapagliflozin) used to treat diabetes, salt-wasting nephropathies such as renal tubular acidosis, polycystic kidney disease and obstructive uropathy, medications like cyclosporine and cisplatin,[1] or conditions like sepsis.[2] Other medications that can cause hyponatremia include oxcarbazepine, trimethoprim, antipsychotics, antidepressants, NSAIDs, cyclophosphamide, carbamazepine, vincristine and vinblastine, thiothixene, thioridazine, other phenothiazines, haloperidol, amitriptyline, other tricyclic antidepressants, monoamine oxidase inhibitors, bromocriptine, clofibrate, general anesthesia, narcotics, opiates, ecstasy, sulfonylureas, and amiodarone.[3]

SALT CONTENT OF FAVORITE FOODS

You can check the salt content on the label of your favorite foods to give yourself a sense of how much salt you're craving—this is useful information for getting acquainted with your salt thermostat—but don't count milligrams per day. Your body will guide you to the right intake. The following list provides the salt content of some common foods.

Food	Sodium Content
Frozen dinners	Up to 1,800 mg per meal
Canned soups and vegetables	Up to 1,300 mg per serving
Cottage cheese	~1,000 mg per cup
Spaghetti sauce	Up to 1,000 mg per cup
Sandwiches	Up to 900 mg per sandwich
Pickles	Up to 785 mg per pickle
Instant beef noodle soup	757 mg per packet
Roasted and salted pumpkin seeds	Up to 711 mg per ounce
Hot dog	Up to 700 mg per hot dog
Tomato juice	Up to 700 mg per 8 ounces
Teriyaki sauce	690 mg per tablespoon
Roquefort cheese	507 mg per ounce

Pretzels	480 mg per ounce
Bagel	~460 mg per bagel
Veggie burger	400–500 mg per patty
Soy sauce	409 mg per teaspoon
American cheese	400 mg per ounce
Salad dressing	Up to 300 mg per 2 tablespoons
Capers	255 mg per tablespoon
6-inch tortilla	~200 mg
Cereal	180 to 300 mg per serving
Cured bacon	175 mg per slice
Ketchup	150 mg per tablespoon
Spinach	125 mg per cup
Sweet relish	122 mg per tablespoon
Beets	65 mg per beet
Celery	50 mg per large stalk of celery
Carrot	50 mg per large carrot

References: http://www.health.com/health/gallery/#cottage-cheese-1;
https://www.healthaliciousness.com/articles/what-foods-high-sodium.php;
http://www.everydayhealth.com/heart-health-pictures/10-sneaky-sodium-bombs.aspx#02;
http://www.webmd.com/diet/ss/slideshow-salt-shockers; and
http://www.foxnews.com/leisure/2013/02/25/8-high-sodium-foods-that-are-ok-to-eat/.

NOTES

. . . .

INTRODUCTION: DON'T FEAR THE SHAKER

1. http://www.cdc.gov/mmwr/preview/mmwrhtml/mm6425a3.htm.

CHAPTER 1: BUT DOESN'T SALT CAUSE HIGH BLOOD PRESSURE?

1. Bayer, R., D. M. Johns, and S. Galea. 2012. Salt and public health: contested science and the challenge of evidence-based decision making. *Health Aff (Millwood)* 31(12): 2738–2746.

2. Overlack, A., et al. 1993. Divergent hemodynamic and hormonal responses to varying salt intake in normotensive subjects. *Hypertension* 22(3): 331–338.

3. Taubes, G. 2007. *Good Calories, Bad Calories.* New York: Knopf.

CHAPTER 2: WE ARE SALTY FOLK

1. Denton, D. A. 1965. Evolutionary aspects of the emergence of aldosterone secretion and salt appetite. *Physiol Rev* 45: 245–295.

2. http://see-the-sea.org/facts/facts-body.htm.

3. https://web.stanford.edu/group/Urchin/mineral.html.

4. http://water.usgs.gov/edu/whyoceansalty.html.

5. Denton, D. A., M. J. McKinley, and R. S. Weisinger. 1996. Hypothalamic integration of body fluid regulation. *Proc Natl Acad Sci U S A* 93(14): 7397–7404.

6. Denton. Evolutionary aspects of the emergence of aldosterone secretion and salt appetite. 245–295.

7. Denton, McKinley, and Weisinger. Hypothalamic integration of body fluid regulation. 7397–7404.

8. Denton, McKinley, and Weisinger. Evolutionary aspects of the emergence of aldosterone secretion and salt appetite. 245–295.

9. http://www.independent.co.uk/news/science/did-humans-come -from-the-seas-instead-of-the-trees-much-derided-theory-of -evolution-about-aquatic-8608288.html; https://answersingenesis.org /natural-selection/adaptation/did-humans-evolve-from-a-fish-out-of -water/; http://evolution.berkeley.edu/evolibrary/article/evograms_04; https://en.m.wikipedia.org/wiki/Evolution_of_tetrapods.

10. Denton. Evolutionary aspects of the emergence of aldosterone secretion and salt appetite. 245–295.

11. Ibid.

12. https://answersingenesis.org/natural-selection/adaptation/did -humans-evolve-from-a-fish-out-of-water/; https://en.m.wikipedia.org /wiki/Evolution_of_tetrapods; https://en.wikipedia.org/wiki/Tetrapod.

13. Denton. Evolutionary aspects of the emergence of aldosterone secretion and salt appetite. 245–295.

14. Ibid.

15. Ibid.

16. Denton, McKinley, and Weisinger. Hypothalamic integration of body fluid regulation. 7397–7404.

17. http://www.scientificamerican.com/article/how-can-sea-mammals -drink/.

18. Luft, F. C., et al. 1979. Plasma and urinary norepinephrine values at extremes of sodium intake in normal man. *Hypertension* 1(3): 261–266.

19. Russon, A. E., et al. 2014. Orangutan fish eating, primate aquatic fauna eating, and their implications for the origins of ancestral hominin fish eating. *J Hum Evol* 77: 50–63.

20. Denton, McKinley, and Weisinger. Hypothalamic integration of body fluid regulation. 7397–7404.

21. Russon. Orangutan fish eating, primate aquatic fauna eating, and their implications for the origins of ancestral hominin fish eating. 50–63.

22. Ibid.

23. Ibid.

24. Ibid.

25. Ibid.

26. Stewart, K. M. 2014. Environmental change and hominin exploitation of C4-based resources in wetland/savanna mosaics. *J Hum Evol* 77: 1–16.

27. Brenna, J. T., and S. E. Carlson. 2014. Docosahexaenoic acid and human brain development: evidence that a dietary supply is needed for optimal development. *J Hum Evol* 77: 99–106.

28. Ibid.

29. http://www.dailymail.co.uk/sciencetech/article-2536015/Ancient -ancestors-ate-diet-tiger-nuts-worms-grasshoppers.html.

30. Agbaje, R. B., V. O. Oyetayo, and A. O. Ojokoh. 2015. Effect of fermentation methods on the mineral, amino and fatty acids composition of *Cyperus esculentus*. *Afr J Biochem Res* 9(7): 89–94.

31. Payne, C. L., et al. 2016. Are edible insects more or less 'healthy' than commonly consumed meats? A comparison using two nutrient profiling models developed to combat over- and undernutrition. *Eur J Clin Nutr* 70(3): 285–291.

32. Xiao, K., et al. 2010. Effects of dietary sodium on performance, flight and compensation strategies in the cotton bollworm, *Helicoverpa armigera* (Hübner) (Lepidoptera: Noctuidae). *Front Zool* 7(11): 1–8.

33. Ibid.

34. Payne. Are edible insects more or less 'healthy' than commonly consumed meats? A comparison using two nutrient profiling models developed to combat over- and undernutrition. 285–291.

35. Meneely, G. R., and H. D. Battarbee. 1976. High sodium-low potassium environment and hypertension. *Am J Cardiol* 38(6): 768–785; Neal, B. 2014. Dietary salt is a public health hazard that requires vigorous attack. *Can J Cardiol* 30(5): 502–506.

36. Eaton, S. B., and M. Konner. 1985. Paleolithic nutrition. A consideration of its nature and current implications. *N Engl J Med* 312(5): 283–289.

37. Denton, D. 1997. Can hypertension be prevented? *J Hum Hypertens* 11(9): 563–569.

38. Gleibermann, L. 1973. Blood pressure and dietary salt in human populations. *Ecol Food Nutr* 2(2): 143–156.

39. O'Keefe, J. H., Jr., and L. Cordain 2004. Cardiovascular disease resulting from a diet and lifestyle at odds with our Paleolithic genome: how to become a 21st-century hunter-gatherer. *Mayo Clin Proc* 79(1): 101–108.

40. Denton. Evolutionary aspects of the emergence of aldosterone secretion and salt appetite. 245–295.

41. Denton, McKinley, and Weisinger. Hypothalamic integration of body fluid regulation. 7397–7404.

42. Folkow, B. 2003. [Salt and blood pressure—centenarian bone of contention]. *Lakartidningen* 100(40): 3142–3147. [Article in Swedish.]

43. Ibid.

44. Milligan, L. P., and B. W. McBride. 1985. Energy costs of ion pumping by animal tissues. *J Nutr* 115(10): 1374–1382.

45. Folkow. [Salt and blood pressure—centenarian bone of contention]. 3142–3147.

46. Overlack, A., et al. 1993. Divergent hemodynamic and hormonal responses to varying salt intake in normotensive subjects. *Hypertension* 22(3): 331–338.

47. Ritz, E. 1996. The history of salt—aspects of interest to the nephrologist. *Nephrol Dial Transplant* 11(6): 969–975.

48. Moinier, B. M., and T. B. Drueke. 2008. Aphrodite, sex and salt—from butterfly to man. *Nephrol Dial Transplant* 23(7): 2154–2161.

49. Ibid.

50. Ibid.

51. Ibid.

52. Denton, McKinley, and Weisinger. Hypothalamic integration of body fluid regulation. 7397–7404.

53. Ritz. The history of salt—aspects of interest to the nephrologist. 969–975.

54. https://en.wikipedia.org/wiki/Mud-puddling.

55. Moinier and Drueke. Aphrodite, sex and salt—from butterfly to man. 2154–2161.

56. Ibid.

57. Wassertheil-Smoller, S., et al. 1991. Effect of antihypertensives on sexual function and quality of life: the TAIM Study. *Ann Intern Med* 114(8): 613–620.

58. Jaaskelainen, J., A. Tiitinen, and R. Voutilainen. 2001. Sexual function and fertility in adult females and males with congenital adrenal hyperplasia. *Horm Res* 56(3–4): 73–80.

CHAPTER 3: THE WAR AGAINST SALT—AND HOW WE DEMONIZED THE WRONG WHITE CRYSTAL

1. Meneely, G. R., and H. D. Battarbee. 1976. High sodium-low potassium environment and hypertension. *Am J Cardiol* 38(6): 768–785; Dahl, L. K. 2005. Possible role of salt intake in the development of essential hypertension. 1960. *Int J Epidemiol* 34(5): 967–972; discussion 972–974, 975–978.

2. Ha, S. K. 2014. Dietary salt intake and hypertension. *Electrolyte Blood Press* 12(1): 7–18.

3. Kurlansky, M. 2003. *Salt: A World History*. New York: Penguin.

4. Ibid.

5. Ibid.

6. Ibid.

7. Mente, A., M. J. O'Donnell, and S. Yusuf. 2014. The population risks of dietary salt excess are exaggerated. *Can J Cardiol* 30(5): 507–512.

8. Ritz, E. 1996. The history of salt—aspects of interest to the nephrologist. *Nephrol Dial Transplant* 11(6): 969–975.

9. Johnson, R. J. 2012. *The Fat Switch*. Mercola.com.

10. Johnson, R. J., et al. 2007. Potential role of sugar (fructose) in the epidemic of hypertension, obesity and the metabolic syndrome, diabetes, kidney disease, and cardiovascular disease. *Am J Clin Nutr* 86(4): 899–906.

11. http://www.heart.org/idc/groups/heart-public/@wcm/@sop/@smd/documents/downloadable/ucm_462020.pdf.

12. http://www.cdc.gov/nchs/data/databriefs/db133.htm; http://www.cdc.gov/mmwr/preview/mmwrhtml/su6203a24.htm.

13. DiNicolantonio, J. J., and S. C. Lucan. 2014. The wrong white crystals: not salt but sugar as aetiological in hypertension and cardiometabolic disease. *Open Heart* 1. doi:10.1136/openhrt-2014-000167.

14. Kurlansky. *Salt: A World History*.

15. Johnson. *The Fat Switch*.

16. Graudal, N. 2005. Commentary: possible role of salt intake in the development of essential hypertension. *Int J Epidemiol* 34: 972–974.

17. Ibid; https://books.google.com/books?id=SFUcAQAAMAAJ&pg=PA652&dq=ambard+lowenstein+salt+1907&hl=en&sa=X&ved=0ahUKEwig-p-9vKvPAhWCcD4KHUjKDoQQ6AEIHDAA#v=onepage&q=lowenstein&f=false; https://books.google.com/books?id=pTTQAAAAMAAJ&pg=PA417&lpg=PA417&dq=lowenstein+salt+1907&source=bl&ots=6hE8bSq3YD&sig=WIq6enQsoTnJaDiL_ZN72y7N2Ew&hl=en&sa=X&ved=0ahUKEwi2xsTt4arPAhXJzIMKHWHOAboQ6AEIIDAB#v=onepage&q=lowenstein%20salt%201907&f=false.

18. Chapman, C. B., and T. B. Gibbons. 1950. The diet and hypertension: a review. *Medicine (Baltimore)* 29(1): 29–69.

19. Ibid; Pines, K. L., and G. A. Perera. 1949. Sodium chloride restriction in hypertensive vascular disease. *Med Clin North Am* 33(3): 713–725.

20. Chasis, H., et al. 1950. Salt and protein restriction: effects on blood pressure and renal hemodynamics in hypertensive patients. *JAMA* 142(10): 711–715.

21. Chapman and Gibbons. The diet and hypertension: a review. 29–69.

22. Klemmer, P., C. E. Grim, and F. C. Luft. 2014. Who and what drove Walter Kempner? The Rice Diet revisited. *Hypertension* 64(4): 684–688.

23. https://en.wikipedia.org/wiki/Rice_diet.

24. Kempner, W. 1948. Treatment of hypertensive vascular disease with Rice Diet. *Am J Med* 4(4): 545–577.

25. Klemmer, Grim, and Luft. Who and what drove Walter Kempner? The Rice Diet revisited. 684–688.

26. Kempner. Treatment of hypertensive vascular disease with Rice Diet. 545–577.

27. Ibid.

28. Batuman, V. 2011. Salt and hypertension: why is there still a debate? *Kidney Int Suppl* 3(4): 316–320.

29. Ratliff, N. B. 2000. Of rice, grain, and zeal: lessons from Drs. Kempner and Esselstyn. *Cleve Clin J Med* 67(8): 565–566.

30. https://news.google.com/newspapers?nid=1955&dat=19971021&id =mEkwAAAAIBAJ&sjid=nKYFAAAAIBAJ&pg=3810,3940249& hl=en.

31. Kempner. Treatment of hypertensive vascular disease with Rice Diet. 545–577.

32. Ibid.

33. McCallum, L., et al. 2013. Serum chloride is an independent predictor of mortality in hypertensive patients. *Hypertension* 62(5): 836–843.

34. Kempner. Treatment of hypertensive vascular disease with Rice Diet. 545–577.

35. http://www.turner-white.com/memberfile.php?PubCode=hp_mar07 _hypertensive.pdf.

36. Kempner. Treatment of hypertensive vascular disease with Rice Diet. 545–577.

37. Chasis. Salt and protein restriction: effects on blood pressure and renal hemodynamics in hypertensive patients. 711–715.

38. Rice Diet in hypertension. *Lancet.* 1950. 256(6637): 529–530.

39. Chasis. Salt and protein restriction: effects on blood pressure and renal hemodynamics in hypertensive patients. 711–715; Laragh, J. H., and M. S. Pecker. 1983. Dietary sodium and essential hypertension:

some myths, hopes, and truths. *Ann Intern Med* 98(5 Pt 2): 735–743; Loofbourow, D. G., A. L. Galbraith, and R. S. Palmer. 1949. Effect of the Rice Diet on the level of the blood pressure in essential hypertension. *N Engl J Med* 240(23): 910–914; Schroeder, H. A., et al. 1949. Low sodium chloride diets in hypertension: effects on blood pressure. *JAMA* 140(5): 458–463; Corcoran, A. C., R. D. Taylor, and I. H. Page. 1951. Controlled observations on the effect of low sodium dietotherapy in essential hypertension. *Circulation* 3(1): 1–16.

40. Laragh and Pecker. Dietary sodium and essential hypertension: some myths, hopes, and truths. 735–743; Loofbourow, Galbraith, and Palmer. Effect of the Rice Diet on the level of the blood pressure in essential hypertension. 910–914; Schroeder. Low sodium chloride diets in hypertension: effects on blood pressure. 458–463; Watkin, D. M., et al. 1950. Effects of diet in essential hypertension. II. Results with unmodified Kempner Rice Diet in 50 hospitalized patients. *Am J Med* 9(4): 441–493; Page, I. H. 1951. Treatment of essential and malignant hypertension. *JAMA* 147(14): 1311–1318.

41. Laragh and Pecker. Dietary sodium and essential hypertension: some myths, hopes, and truths. 735–743.

42. Ibid; Reisin, E., et al. 1978. Effect of weight loss without salt restriction on the reduction of blood pressure in overweight hypertensive patients. *N Engl J Med* 298(1): 1–6; Tuck, M. L., et al. 1981. The effect of weight reduction on blood pressure, plasma renin activity, and plasma aldosterone levels in obese patients. *N Engl J Med* 304(16): 930–933.

43. Corcoran, Taylor, and Page. Controlled observations on the effect of low sodium dietotherapy in essential hypertension. 1–16.

44. Loofbourow, Galbraith, and Palmer. Effect of the Rice Diet on the level of the blood pressure in essential hypertension. 910–914.

45. Tasdemir, V., et al. 2015. Hyponatremia in the outpatient setting: clinical characteristics, risk factors, and outcome. *Int Urol Nephrol* 47(12): 1977–1983.

46. Laragh and Pecker. Dietary sodium and essential hypertension: some myths, hopes, and truths. 735–743; Mac, G. W., Jr. 1948. Risk of uremia due to sodium depletion. *JAMA* 137(16): 1377; Soloff, L. A., and J. Zatuchni, 1949. Syndrome of salt depletion induced by a regimen of sodium restriction and sodium diuresis. *JAMA* 139(17): 1136–1139; Grollman, A. R., et al. 1945. Sodium restriction in the diet for hypertension. *JAMA* 129(8): 533–537.

47. Schroeder. Low sodium chloride diets in hypertension: effects on blood pressure. 458–463.

48. Joe, B. 2015. Dr Lewis Kitchener Dahl, the Dahl rats, and the "inconvenient truth" about the genetics of hypertension. *Hypertension* 65(5): 963–969.

49. Dahl. Possible role of salt intake in the development of essential hypertension. 967–972; discussion 972–974, 975–978.

50. Joe. Dr Lewis Kitchener Dahl, the Dahl rats, and the "inconvenient truth" about the genetics of hypertension. 963–969.

51. Dahl, L. K., and R. A. Love. 1954. Evidence for relationship between sodium (chloride) intake and human essential hypertension. *AMA Arch Intern Med* 94(4): 525–531.

52. Rebello, T., R. E. Hodges, and J. L. Smith. 1983. Short-term effects of various sugars on antinatriuresis and blood pressure changes in normotensive young men. *Am J Clin Nutr* 38(1): 84–94.

53. Kearns, C. E., L. A. Schmidt, and S. A. Glantz. 2016. Sugar industry and coronary heart disease research: a historical analysis of internal industry documents. *JAMA Intern Med* 176(11): 1680–1685.

54. Dahl. Possible role of salt intake in the development of essential hypertension. 967–972; discussion 972–974, 975–978.

55. Ibid.

56. Folkow, B., and D. L. Ely. 1987. Dietary sodium effects on cardiovascular and sympathetic neuroeffector functions as studied in various rat models. *J Hypertens* 5(4): 383–395.

57. Grollman. Sodium restriction in the diet for hypertension. 533–537.

58. Dahl, L. K. 1968. Salt in processed baby foods. *Am J Clin Nutr* 21(8): 787–792; Infant mortality in the United States and abroad. *Stat Bull Metropol Life Insur Co*, 1967. 48: 2–6.

59. Dahl. Salt in processed baby foods. 787–792.

60. Meneely, G. R., and H. D. Battarbee. 1976. High sodium-low potassium environment and hypertension. *Am J Cardiol* 38(6): 768–785.

61. https://thescienceofnutrition.files.wordpress.com/2014/03/dietary-goals-for-the-united-states.pdf.

62. http://www.nytimes.com/1987/09/20/obituaries/george-r-meneely-75-dies-louisiana-medical-professor.html.

63. Meneely and Battarbee. High sodium-low potassium environment and hypertension. 768–785.

64. http://babel.hathitrust.org/cgi/pt?id=umn.31951d00283417h;view=1up;seq=7.

65. http://zerodisease.com/archive/Dietary_Goals_For_The_United_States.pdf.

66. http://babel.hathitrust.org/cgi/pt?id=umn.31951d00283417h;view=1up;seq=7.

67. Meneely and Battarbee. High sodium-low potassium environment and hypertension. 768–785.

68. http://babel.hathitrust.org/cgi/pt?id=umn.31951d00283417h;view=1up;seq=7.

69. Pearce, E. N., M. Andersson, and M. B. Zimmermann. 2013. Global iodine nutrition: where do we stand in 2013? *Thyroid* 23(5): 523–528.

70. Brown, W. J., Jr., F. K. Brown, and I. Krishan. 1971. Exchangeable sodium and blood volume in normotensive and hypertensive humans on high and low sodium intake. *Circulation* 43(4): 508–519.

71. Luft, F. C., et al. 1979. Plasma and urinary norepinephrine values at extremes of sodium intake in normal man. *Hypertension* 1(3): 261–266; Grant, H., and F. Reischsman. 1946. The effects of the ingestion of large amounts of sodium chloride on the arterial and venous pressures of normal subjects. *Am Heart J* 32(6): 704–712; Kirkendall, A. M., et al. 1976. The effect of dietary sodium chloride on blood pressure, body fluids, electrolytes, renal function, and serum lipids of normotensive man. *J Lab Clin Med* 87(3): 411–434.

72. Guyton, A. C., et al. 1980. Salt balance and long-term blood pressure control. *Annu Rev Med* 31: 15–27.

73. Luft. Plasma and urinary norepinephrine values at extremes of sodium intake in normal man. 261–266.

74. DiNicolantonio and Lucan. The wrong white crystals: not salt but sugar as aetiological in hypertension and cardiometabolic disease; Johnson, R. J., et al. 2015. The discovery of hypertension: evolving views on the role of the kidneys, and current hot topics. *Am J Physiol Renal Physiol* 308(3): F167–F178.

75. Meneely and Battarbee. High sodium-low potassium environment and hypertension. 768–785.

76. Loofbourow, Galbraith, and Palmer. Effect of the Rice Diet on the level of the blood pressure in essential hypertension. 910–914.

77. Dahl. Possible role of salt intake in the development of essential hypertension. 967–972; discussion 972–974, 975–978.

78. http://www.legacy.com/obituaries/nytimes/obituary.aspx?pid=174460411.

79. Laragh and Pecker. Dietary sodium and essential hypertension: some myths, hopes, and truths. 735–743.

80. MacGregor, G. A., et al. 1982. Double-blind randomised crossover trial of moderate sodium restriction in essential hypertension. *Lancet* 1(8268): 351–355.

81. http://www.health.gov/dietaryguidelines/dga2010/dietaryguidelines 2010.pdf.

82. http://www.actiononsalt.org.uk/about/Staff Profiles/42511.html.

83. http://www.worldactiononsalt.com/about/index.html.

84. http://www.actiononsalt.org.uk/news/Salt in the news/2014/126738 .html.

85. Law, M. R., C. D. Frost, and N. J. Wald. 1991. By how much does dietary salt reduction lower blood pressure? III—Analysis of data from trials of salt reduction. *BMJ* 302(6780): 819–824.

86. Graudal, N. A., A. M. Galloe, and P. Garred. 1998. Effects of sodium restriction on blood pressure, renin, aldosterone, catecholamines, cholesterols, and triglyceride: a meta-analysis. *JAMA* 279(17): 1383–1391; Midgley, J. P., et al. 1996. Effect of reduced dietary sodium on blood pressure: a meta-analysis of randomized controlled trials. *JAMA* 275(20): 1590–1597.

87. The fifth report of the Joint National Committee on Detection, Evaluation, and Treatment of High Blood Pressure (JNC V). *Arch Intern Med.* 1993. 153(2): 154–183.

88. Swales, J. 2000. Population advice on salt restriction: the social issues. *Am J Hypertens* 13(1 Pt 1): 2–7.

89. Ibid.

90. Graudal, Galloe, and Garred. Effects of sodium restriction on blood pressure, renin, aldosterone, catecholamines, cholesterols, and triglyceride: a meta-analysis. 1383–1391; Midgley. Effect of reduced dietary sodium on blood pressure: a meta-analysis of randomized controlled trials. 1590–1597; Swales, J. D. 1995. Dietary sodium restriction in hypertension. In J. H. Laragh and B. M. Brenner, eds., *Hypertension: Pathophysiology, Diagnosis and Management,* 283–298. New York: Raven Press.

91. Cutler, J. A., D. Follmann, and S. Allender. 1997. Randomized trials of sodium reduction: an overview. *Am J Clin Nutr* 65(2 Suppl): 643s–651s.

92. Kumanyika, S. K., et al. 1993. Feasibility and efficacy of sodium reduction in the Trials of Hypertension Prevention, phase I. Trials of Hypertension Prevention Collaborative Research Group. *Hypertension* 22(4): 502–512.

93. Ebrahim, S., and G. D. Smith. 1998. Lowering blood pressure: a systematic review of sustained effects of non-pharmacological interventions. *J Public Health Med* 20(4): 441–448.

94. Swales, J. D. 1991. Dietary salt and blood pressure: the role of meta-analyses. *J Hypertens Suppl* 9(6): S42–S46; discussion S47–S49.

95. Midgley. Effect of reduced dietary sodium on blood pressure: a meta-analysis of randomized controlled trials. 1590–1597.

96. Food and Nutrition Board. 1989. *Diet and Health: Implications for Reducing Chronic Disease Risk.* Washington, DC: National Academies Press; King, J. C., and K. J. Reimers. 2014. Beyond blood pressure: new paradigms in sodium intake reduction and health outcomes. *Adv Nutr* 5(5): 550–552; Sodium, potassium, body mass, alcohol and blood pressure: the INTERSALT Study. The INTERSALT Co-operative Research Group. *J Hypertens Suppl.* 1988. 6(4): S584–S586.

97. Intersalt: an international study of electrolyte excretion and blood pressure. Results for 24 hour urinary sodium and potassium excretion. Intersalt Cooperative Research Group. *BMJ.* 1988. 297(6644): 319–328.

98. Folkow, B., and D. Ely. 1998. Importance of the blood pressure-heart rate relationship. *Blood Press* 7(3): 133–138.

99. Overlack, A., et al. 1993. Divergent hemodynamic and hormonal responses to varying salt intake in normotensive subjects. *Hypertension* 22(3): 331–338.

100. Freedman, D. A., and D. B. Petitti. 2001. Salt and blood pressure. Conventional wisdom reconsidered. *Eval Rev* 25(3): 267–287.

101. Folkow, B. 2003. [Salt and blood pressure—centenarian bone of contention]. *Lakartidningen* 100(40): 3142–3147. [Article in Swedish.]; Folkow and Ely. Importance of the blood pressure-heart rate relationship. 133–138.

102. Food and Nutrition Board. 2005. Dietary Reference Intakes for Water, Potassium, Sodium, Chloride, and Sulfate By Standing Committee on the Scientific Evaluation of Dietary Reference Intakes, Panel on Dietary Reference Intakes for Electrolytes and Water. Washington, DC: Institute of Medicine.

103. Ibid.

104. Ibid.

105. http://www.health.gov/dietaryguidelines/dga2005/document/pdf/dga2005.pdf.

106. http://www.jhsph.edu/faculty/directory/profile/15/lawrence-j-appel.

107. http://www.nap.edu/read/10925/chapter/1%20-%20ov.

108. http://www.worldactiononsalt.com/about/members/index.html.

109. http://www.health.gov/dietaryguidelines/dga2010/dietaryguidelines 2010.pdf.

110. http://www.forbes.com/sites/realspin/2015/04/09/if-you-must-have-a-dietary-culprit-at-least-pick-the-right-one/.

111. Dietary fat and its relation to heart attacks and strokes. Report by the Central Committee for Medical and Community Program of the American Heart Association. JAMA 175(5): 389–391.

112. http://garytaubes.com/wp-content/uploads/2011/08/science-political-science-of-salt.pdf.

113. http://www.theguardian.com/society/2003/apr/21/usnews.food.

114. http://www.thedrum.com/news/2016/07/20/coca-cola-use-olympics-sponsorship-push-non-fizzy-drinks; http://fluoridealert.org/news/sugar-industry-has-subverted-public-health-policy-for-decades-study-finds/.

115. http://well.blogs.nytimes.com/2015/08/09/coca-cola-funds-scientists-who-shift-blame-for-obesity-away-from-bad-diets/?_r=0; http://www.eurekalert.org/pub_releases/2015-02/bmj-bir020915.php; http://www.naturalnews.com/049027_Coca-Cola_payola_scheme_corporate_propaganda.html; http://finance.yahoo.com/news/coke-healthy-snack-company-gets-message-104133830.html.

116. Lucan, S. C., and J. J. DiNicolantonio. 2015. How calorie-focused thinking about obesity and related diseases may mislead and harm public health. An alternative. Public Health Nutr 18(4): 571–581.

117. Walker, A. R. 1975. Sucrose, hypertension, and heart disease. Am J Clin Nutr 28(3): 195–200.

118. Sievenpiper, J. L., L. Tappy, and F. Brouns. 2015. Letter to the editor regarding: DiNicolantonio JJ, O'Keefe JH, Lucan SC. Added Fructose: A Principal Driver of Type 2 Diabetes Mellitus and Its Consequences. Mayo Clin Proc January 26. pii: S0025-6196(15)00040-3. doi:10.1016/j.mayocp.2014.12.019. [Epub ahead of print] Review.

119. Johnson. Potential role of sugar (fructose) in the epidemic of hypertension, obesity and the metabolic syndrome, diabetes, kidney disease, and cardiovascular disease. 899–906; DiNicolantonio and Lucan. The wrong white crystals: not salt but sugar as aetiological in hypertension and cardiometabolic disease; DiNicolantonio, J. J., J. H. O'Keefe, and S. C. Lucan. 2015. In reply—fructose as a driver of diabetes: an incomplete view of the evidence. Mayo Clin Proc 90(7): 988–990; DiNicolantonio, J. J., J. H. O'Keefe, and S. C. Lucan. 2014. An unsavory truth: sugar, more than salt, predisposes to hypertension and chronic disease. Am J Cardiol 114(7): 1126–1128; DiNicolantonio, J. J., J. H. O'Keefe, and S. C. Lucan, Added fructose: a principal driver of type 2 diabetes mellitus and its consequences. Mayo Clin Proc 90(3): 372–381; Basu, S., et al. 2013. The relationship of sugar to population-level diabetes prevalence: an econometric analysis of repeated cross-sectional data. PLoS One 8(2): e57873.

120. http://zerodisease.com/archive/Dietary_Goals_For_The_United_States.pdf.

121. https://thescienceofnutrition.files.wordpress.com/2014/03/dietary
     -goals-for-the-united-states.pdf.

122. http://content.time.com/time/covers/0,16641,19820315,00.html.

123. http://content.time.com/time/covers/0,16641,19840326,00.html.

124. http://content.time.com/time/covers/0,16641,19610113,00.html.

125. http://www.health.gov/dietaryguidelines/1980thin.pdf;   http://www
     .health.gov/dietaryguidelines/1985thin.pdf;   http://www.health.gov
     /dietaryguidelines/1990thin.pdf; http://www.cnpp.usda.gov/sites/default
     /files/dietary_guidelines_for_americans/1995DGConsumerBrochure
     .pdf.

126. Rebello, Hodges, and Smith. Short-term effects of various sugars on
     antinatriuresis and blood pressure changes in normotensive young
     men. 84–94; Reiser, S., et al. 1981. Serum insulin and glucose in hy-
     perinsulinemic subjects fed three different levels of sucrose. *Am J Clin
     Nutr* 34(11): 2348–2358; Yudkin, J. 1964. Patterns and trends in car-
     bohydrate consumption and their relation to disease. *Proc Nutr Soc*
     23: 149–162; Yudkin, J. 1964. Dietary fat and dietary sugar in relation
     to ischaemic heart-disease and diabetes. *Lancet* 2(7349): 4–5.

127. Reiser, S., et al. 1979. Isocaloric exchange of dietary starch and su-
     crose in humans. II. Effect on fasting blood insulin, glucose, and glu-
     cagon and on insulin and glucose response to a sucrose load. *Am J
     Clin Nutr* 32(11): 2206–2216.

128. Reiser. Serum insulin and glucose in hyperinsulinemic subjects fed
     three different levels of sucrose. 2348–2358.

129. DiNicolantonio, O'Keefe, and Lucan. Added fructose: a principal
     driver of type 2 diabetes mellitus and its consequences. 372–381.

130. Hujoel, P. 2009. Dietary carbohydrates and dental-systemic diseases.
     J Dent Res 88(6): 490–502.

131. Bes-Rastrollo, M., et al. 2013. Financial conflicts of interest and re-
     porting bias regarding the association between sugar-sweetened bev-
     erages and weight gain: a systematic review of systematic reviews.
     PLoS Med 10(12): e1001578; discussion e1001578.

132. http://www.youtube.com/watch?v=eIIaGlBVphI.

133. Bray, G. A., and B. M. Popkin. 2014. Dietary sugar and body weight:
     have we reached a crisis in the epidemic of obesity and diabetes?
     Health be damned! Pour on the sugar. *Diabetes Care* 37(4): 950–956.

134. https://thescienceofnutrition.files.wordpress.com/2014/03/dietary
     -goals-for-the-united-states.pdf.

135. Johnson. Potential role of sugar (fructose) in the epidemic of hyper-
     tension, obesity and the metabolic syndrome, diabetes, kidney dis-
     ease, and cardiovascular disease. 899–906.

136. Bernstein, A. M., and W. C. Willett. 2010. Trends in 24-h urinary sodium excretion in the United States, 1957–2003: a systematic review. *Am J Clin Nutr* 92(5): 1172–1180.

137. DiNicolantonio and Lucan. The wrong white crystals: not salt but sugar as aetiological in hypertension and cardiometabolic disease; http://www.ers.usda.gov/data-products/food-availability-(per-capita) -data-system/food-availability-documentation.aspx).

138. http://www.qmfound.com/history_of_rations.htm.

139. http://www.qmfound.com/army_rations_historical_background.htm.

140. Ibid.

141. https://en.wikipedia.org/wiki/Refrigeration.

142. http://www.cdc.gov/nchs/data/databriefs/db88.pdf.

143. Antar, M. A., M. A. Ohlson, and R. E. Hodges. Changes in retail market food supplies in the United States in the last seventy years in relation to the incidence of coronary heart disease, with special reference to dietary carbohydrates and essential fatty acids. *Am J Clin Nutr* 14: 169–178.

144. http://health.gov/dietaryguidelines/2015-scientific-report/pdfs /scientific-report-of-the-2015-dietary-guidelines-advisory-committee .pdf.

145. http://www.health.gov/dietaryguidelines/1980thin.pdf.

146. Trumbo, P., et al. 2002. Dietary reference intakes for energy, carbohydrate, fiber, fat, fatty acids, cholesterol, protein and amino acids. *J Am Diet Assoc* 102(11): 1621–1630.

147. http://www.health.gov/dietaryguidelines/dga2005/document/pdf /dga2005.pdf.

148. http://www.health.gov/dietaryguidelines/dga2010/dietaryguidelines 2010.pdf.

149. http://health.gov/dietaryguidelines/2015-scientific-report/pdfs /scientific-report-of-the-2015-dietary-guidelines-advisory-committee .pdf.

CHAPTER 4: WHAT *REALLY* CAUSES HEART DISEASE?

1. Park, J., and C. K. Kwock. 2015. Sodium intake and prevalence of hypertension, coronary heart disease, and stroke in Korean adults. *J Ethn Foods* 2(3): 92–96.

2. http://www.worldlifeexpectancy.com/cause-of-death/coronary-heart -disease/by-country/).

3. http://ec.europa.eu/health/nutrition_physical_activity/docs/salt _report1_en.pdf.

4. http://www.worldlifeexpectancy.com/cause-of-death/coronary-heart -disease/by-country/).

5. https://en.wikipedia.org/wiki/List_of_countries_by_life_expectancy.

6. http://ec.europa.eu/health/nutrition_physical_activity/docs/salt _report1_en.pdf; http://ec.europa.eu/eurostat/statistics-explained/index .php/Causes_of_death_statistics; Elliot, P., and I. Brown. 2006. Sodium intakes around the world. http://www.who.int/dietphysical activity/Elliot-brown-2007.pdf.

7. https://en.wikipedia.org/wiki/Kimchi.

8. Park and Kwock. Sodium intake and prevalence of hypertension, coronary heart disease, and stroke in Korean adults. 92–96.

9. Elliot and Brown. Sodium intakes around the world.

10. Timio, M., et al. 1997. Blood pressure trend and cardiovascular events in nuns in a secluded order: a 30-year follow-up study. *Blood Press* 6(2): 81–87.

11. Chappuis, A., et al. 2011. Swiss survey on salt intake: main results. https://serval.unil.ch/resource/serval:BIB%5f16AEF897B618.P001 /REF.

12. Ibid.

13. https://en.wikipedia.org/wiki/List_of_countries_by_life_expectancy.

14. http://ec.europa.eu/health/nutrition_physical_activity/docs/salt _report1_en.pdf; http://ec.europa.eu/eurostat/statistics-explained/index .php/Causes_of_death_statistics; Elliot and Brown. Sodium intakes around the world.

15. Park and Kwock. Sodium intake and prevalence of hypertension, coronary heart disease, and stroke in Korean adults. 92–96.

16. Graudal, N. A., A. M. Galloe, and P. Garred. 1998. Effects of sodium restriction on blood pressure, renin, aldosterone, catecholamines, cholesterols, and triglyceride: a meta-analysis. *JAMA* 279(17): 1383–1391.

17. Ibid.

18. Kotchen, T. A., et al. 1989. Baroreceptor sensitivity in prehypertensive young adults. 13(6 Pt 2): 878–883; Longworth, D. L., et al. 1980. Divergent blood pressure responses during short-term sodium restriction in hypertension. *Clin Pharmacol Ther* 27(4): 544–546; Weinberger, M. H., et al. 1986. Definitions and characteristics of sodium sensitivity and blood pressure resistance. *Hypertension* 8(6 Pt 2): II127–II134; Egan, B. M., et al. 1991. Neurohumoral and metabolic effects of short-term dietary NaCl restriction in men. Relationship to salt-sensitivity status. *Am J Hypertens* 4(5 Pt 1): 416–421.

19. Graudal, Galloe, and Garred. Effects of sodium restriction on blood pressure, renin, aldosterone, catecholamines, cholesterols, and triglyceride: a meta-analysis. 1383–1391.

20. Sullivan, J. M., et al. 1980. Hemodynamic effects of dietary sodium in man: a preliminary report. *Hypertension* 2(4): 506–514.

21. Heaney, R. P. 2015. Making sense of the science of sodium. *Nutr Today* 50(2): 63–66.

22. Ibid.

23. Luft, F. C., et al. 1979. Plasma and urinary norepinephrine values at extremes of sodium intake in normal man. *Hypertension* 1(3): 261–266.

24. McDonough, D. J., and C. M. Wilhelmj. 1954. The effect of excess salt intake on human blood pressure. *Am J Dig Dis* 21(7): 180–181; Murray, R. H., et al. 1978. Blood pressure responses to extremes of sodium intake in normal man. *Proc Soc Exp Biol Med* 159(3): 432–436.

25. Murray. Blood pressure responses to extremes of sodium intake in normal man. 432–436.

26. Luft. Plasma and urinary norepinephrine values at extremes of sodium intake in normal man. 261–266.

27. Kirkendall, A. M., et al. 1976. The effect of dietary sodium chloride on blood pressure, body fluids, electrolytes, renal function, and serum lipids of normotensive man. *J Lab Clin Med* 87(3): 411–434.

28. Scribner, B. H. 1983. Salt and hypertension. *JAMA* 250(3): 388–389.

29. Egan. Neurohumoral and metabolic effects of short-term dietary NaCl restriction in men. Relationship to salt-sensitivity status. 416–421.

30. Longworth. Divergent blood pressure responses during short-term sodium restriction in hypertension. 544–546.

31. Heer, M., et al. 2000. High dietary sodium chloride consumption may not induce body fluid retention in humans. *Am J Physiol Renal Physiol* 278(4): F585–F595.

32. Haddy, F. J., and M. B. Pamnani. 1985. The kidney in the pathogenesis of hypertension: the role of sodium. *Am J Kidney Dis* 5(4): A5–A13; Beretta-Piccoli, C., et al. 1984. Body sodium blood volume state in essential hypertension: abnormal relation of exchangeable sodium to age and blood pressure in male patients. *J Cardiovasc Pharmacol* 6 (Suppl 1): S134–S142.

33. Finnerty, F. A., Jr., et al. 1970. Influence of extracellular fluid volume on response to antihypertensive drugs. *Circ Res* 27(1 Suppl 1): 71–82.

34. Luft. Plasma and urinary norepinephrine values at extremes of sodium intake in normal man. 261–266.

35. Kirkendall. The effect of dietary sodium chloride on blood pressure, body fluids, electrolytes, renal function, and serum lipids of normotensive man. 411–434.

36. Freis, E. D. 1976. Salt, volume and the prevention of hypertension. *Circulation* 53(4): 589–595.

37. Heaney. Making sense of the science of sodium. 63–66.

38. Srinivasan, S. R., et al. 1980. Effects of dietary sodium and sucrose on the induction of hypertension in spider monkeys. *Am J Clin Nutr* 33(3): 561–569.

39. Haddy and Pamnani. The kidney in the pathogenesis of hypertension: the role of sodium. A5–A13.

40. Overlack, A., et al. 1993. Divergent hemodynamic and hormonal responses to varying salt intake in normotensive subjects. *Hypertension* 22(3): 331–338; Folkow, B., and D. Ely. 1998. Importance of the blood pressure-heart rate relationship. *Blood Press* 7(3): 133–138.

41. Folkow, B. 2003. [Salt and blood pressure—centenarian bone of contention]. *Lakartidningen* 100(40): 3142–3147. [Article in Swedish]; Folkow and Ely. Importance of the blood pressure-heart rate relationship. 133–138.

42. Omvik, P., and P. Lund-Johansen. 1986. Is sodium restriction effective treatment of borderline and mild essential hypertension? A long-term haemodynamic study at rest and during exercise. 4(5): 535–541; Omvik, P., and P. Lund-Johansen. Hemodynamic effects at rest and during exercise of long-term sodium restriction in mild essential hypertension. *Acta Med Scand Suppl* 714: 71–74.

43. McCarty, M. F. 2005. Marinobufagenin may mediate the impact of salty diets on left ventricular hypertrophy by disrupting the protective function of coronary microvascular endothelium. *Med Hypotheses* 64(4): 854–863.

44. Ibid; Fedorova, O. V., et al. 2001. Marinobufagenin, an endogenous alpha-1 sodium pump ligand, in hypertensive Dahl salt-sensitive rats. *Hypertension* 37(2 Pt 2): 462–466.

45. Omvik and Lund-Johansen. Is sodium restriction effective treatment of borderline and mild essential hypertension? A long-term haemodynamic study at rest and during exercise. 535–541; Omvik and Lund-Johansen. Hemodynamic effects at rest and during exercise of long-term sodium restriction in mild essential hypertension. 71–74.

46. Bagrov, Y. Y., et al. 2005. Marinobufagenin, an endogenous inhibitor of alpha-1 Na/K-ATPase, is a novel factor in pathogenesis of diabetes mellitus. *Dokl Biol Sci* 404: 333–337; Bagrov, Y. Y., et al. 2005.

Endogenous digitalis-like ligands and Na/K-ATPase inhibition in experimental diabetes mellitus. *Front Biosci* 10: 2257–2262.

47. Bagrov, Y. Y., et al. 2007. Endogenous sodium pump inhibitors, diabetes mellitus and preeclampsia. *Pathophysiol* 14(3–4): 147–151.

48. DiNicolantonio, J. J., J. H. O'Keefe, and S. C. Lucan. Added fructose: a principal driver of type 2 diabetes mellitus and its consequences. *Mayo Clin Proc* 90(3): 372–381.

49. Johnson, R. J., et al. 2007. Potential role of sugar (fructose) in the epidemic of hypertension, obesity and the metabolic syndrome, diabetes, kidney disease, and cardiovascular disease. *Am J Clin Nutr* 86(4): 899–906; Bes-Rastrollo, M., et al. 2013. Financial conflicts of interest and reporting bias regarding the association between sugar-sweetened beverages and weight gain: a systematic review of systematic reviews. *PLoS Med* 10(12): e1001578; discussion e1001578; Nakayama, T., et al. 2010. Dietary fructose causes tubulointerstitial injury in the normal rat kidney. *Am J Physiol Renal Physiol* 298(3): F712–F720; Cirillo, P., et al. 2009. Ketohexokinase-dependent metabolism of fructose induces proinflammatory mediators in proximal tubular cells. *J Am Soc Nephrol* 20(3): 545–553.

50. DiNicolantonio, O'Keefe, and Lucan. Added fructose: a principal driver of type 2 diabetes mellitus and its consequences. 372–381; Basu, S., et al. 2013. The relationship of sugar to population-level diabetes prevalence: an econometric analysis of repeated cross-sectional data. *PLoS One* 8(2): e57873; Reiser, S., et al. 1981. Serum insulin and glucose in hyperinsulinemic subjects fed three different levels of sucrose. *Am J Clin Nutr* 34(11): 2348–2358.

51. Reiser. Serum insulin and glucose in hyperinsulinemic subjects fed three different levels of sucrose. 2348–2358.

52. McCarty. Marinobufagenin may mediate the impact of salty diets on left ventricular hypertrophy by disrupting the protective function of coronary microvascular endothelium. 854–863.

53. Giampietro, O., et al. 1988. Increased urinary excretion of digoxin-like immunoreactive substance by insulin-dependent diabetic patients: a linkage with hypertension? *Clin Chem* 34(12): 2418–2422.

54. Weidmann, P., and B. N. Trost. 1985. Pathogenesis and treatment of hypertension associated with diabetes. *Horm Metab Res Suppl* 15: 51–58; Christlieb, A. R., et al. 1985. Is insulin the link between hypertension and obesity? *Hypertension* 7(6 Pt 2): II54–II57.

55. Weidmann, P., C. Beretta-Piccoli, and B. N. Trost. Pressor factors and responsiveness in hypertension accompanying diabetes mellitus. *Hypertension* 7(6 Pt 2): II33–II42; O'Hare, J. A., et al. 1985. Exchangeable

sodium and renin in hypertensive diabetic patients with and without nephropathy. *Hypertension* 7(6 Pt 2): II43–II48; Feldt-Rasmussen, B., et al. 1987. Central role for sodium in the pathogenesis of blood pressure changes independent of angiotensin, aldosterone and catecholamines in type 1 (insulin-dependent) diabetes mellitus. *Diabetologia* 30(8): 610–617.

56. DeFronzo, R. A. 1981. The effect of insulin on renal sodium metabolism. A review with clinical implications. *Diabetologia* 21(3): 165–171; Vierhapper, H. 1985. Effect of exogenous insulin on blood pressure regulation in healthy and diabetic subjects. *Hypertension* 7(6 Pt 2): II49–II53.

57. Johansen, K., and A. P. Hansen. 1969. High 24-hour level of serum growth hormone in juvenile diabetics. *BMJ* 2(5653): 356–357.

58. Giampietro. Increased urinary excretion of digoxin-like immunoreactive substance by insulin-dependent diabetic patients: a linkage with hypertension? 2418–2422; Deray, G., et al. 1987. Evidence of an endogenous digitalis-like factor in the plasma of patients with acromegaly. *N Engl J Med* 316(10): 575–580.

59. Greene, D. A., S. A. Lattimer, and A. A. Sima. 1987. Sorbitol, phosphoinositides, and sodium-potassium-ATPase in the pathogenesis of diabetic complications. *N Engl J Med* 316(10): 599–606; Das, P. K., et al. 1976. Diminished ouabain-sensitive, sodium-potassium ATPase activity in sciatic nerves of rats with streptozotocin-induced diabetes. *Exp Neurol* 53(1): 285–288; Pierce, G. N., and N. S. Dhalla. 1983. Sarcolemmal Na+-K+-ATPase activity in diabetic rat heart. *Am J Physiol* 245(3): C241–C247; Finotti, P., and P. Palatini. 1986. Reduction of erythrocyte (Na+-K+)ATPase activity in type 1 (insulin-dependent) diabetic subjects and its activation by homologous plasma. *Diabetologia* 29(9): 623–628.

60. Jakobsen, J., G. M. Knudsen, and M. Juhler. Cation permeability of the blood-brain barrier in streptozotocin-diabetic rats. *Diabetologia* 30(6): 409–413; Moore, R. D. 1993. *The High Blood Pressure Solution.* Rochester, VT: Healing Arts Press.

61. Ng, L. L., M. Harker, and E. D. Abel. 1989. Leucocyte sodium content and sodium pump activity in overweight and lean hypertensives. *Clin Endocrinol (Oxf)* 30(2): 191–200.

62. Ferrannini, E., et al. 1989. Hypertension: a metabolic disorder? *Diabetes Metab* 15(5 Pt 2): 284–291; Ferrannini, E., et al. 1987. Insulin resistance in essential hypertension. *N Engl J Med* 317(6): 350–357; Reaven, G. M., and B. B. Hoffman. 1987. A role for insulin in the aetiology and course of hypertension? *Lancet* 2(8556): 435–437.

63. Cambien, F., et al. 1987. Body mass, blood pressure, glucose, and lipids. Does plasma insulin explain their relationships? *Arteriosclerosis* 7(2): 197–202.

64. Christlieb. Is insulin the link between hypertension and obesity? II54–II57; Vasdev, S., and J. Stuckless. 2010. Role of methylglyoxal in essential hypertension. *Int J Angiol* 19(2): e58–e65.

65. Ferrannini. Insulin resistance in essential hypertension. 350–357.

66. Yudkin, J. 1972. Sucrose and cardiovascular disease. *Proc Nutr Soc* 31(3): 331–337; Macdonald, I. 1971. Effects of dietary carbohydrate on lipid metabolism in primates. *Proc Nutr Soc* 30(3): 277–282.

67. Feldman, R. D., A. G. Logan, and N. D. Schmidt. 1996. Dietary salt restriction increases vascular insulin resistance. *Clin Pharmacol Ther* 60(4): 444–451; Feldman, R. D., and N. D. Schmidt. 1999. Moderate dietary salt restriction increases vascular and systemic insulin resistance. *Am J Hypertens* 12(6): 643–647.

68. Yudkin, J., V. V. Kakkar, and S. Szanto. 1969. Sugar intake, serum insulin and platelet adhesiveness in men with and without peripheral vascular disease. *Postgrad Med J* 45(527): 608–611.

69. Pazarloglou, M., et al. 2007. Evaluation of insulin resistance and sodium sensitivity in normotensive offspring of hypertensive individuals. *Am J Kidney Dis* 49(4): 540–546.

70. Ibid.

71. Falkner, B., et al. 1990. Insulin resistance and blood pressure in young black men. *Hypertension* 16(6): 706–711.

72. Pazarloglou. Evaluation of insulin resistance and sodium sensitivity in normotensive offspring of hypertensive individuals. 540–546.

73. Reaven, G. M., H. Lithell, and L. Landsberg. 1996. Hypertension and associated metabolic abnormalities—the role of insulin resistance and the sympathoadrenal system. *N Engl J Med* 334(6): 374–381; Scaglione, R., et al. 1995. Central obesity and hypertension: pathophysiologic role of renal haemodynamics and function. *Int J Obes Relat Metab Disord* 19(6): 403–409.

74. Sharma, A. M., et al. 1991. Salt sensitivity in young normotensive subjects is associated with a hyperinsulinemic response to oral glucose. *J Hypertens* 9(4): 329–335; Zavaroni, I., et al. 1995. Association between salt sensitivity and insulin concentrations in patients with hypertension. *Am J Hypertens* 8(8): 855–858; Fuenmayor, N., E. Moreira, and L. X. Cubeddu. 1998. Salt sensitivity is associated with insulin resistance in essential hypertension. *Am J Hypertens* 11(4 Pt 1): 397–402; Bigazzi, R., et al. 1996. Clustering of cardiovas-

cular risk factors in salt-sensitive patients with essential hypertension: role of insulin. *Am J Hypertens* 9(1): 24–32.

75. Hoffmann, I. S., A. B. Alfieri, and L. X. Cubeddu. 2007. Effects of lifestyle changes and metformin on salt sensitivity and nitric oxide metabolism in obese salt-sensitive Hispanics. *J Hum Hypertens* 21(7): 571–578.

76. Rocchini, A. P., et al. 1989. The effect of weight loss on the sensitivity of blood pressure to sodium in obese adolescents. *N Engl J Med* 321(9): 580–585.

77. Muntzel, M. S., I. Hamidou, and S. Barrett. 1999. Metformin attenuates salt-induced hypertension in spontaneously hypertensive rats. *Hypertension* 33(5): 1135–1140.

78. Muntzel, M. S., B. Nyeduala, and S. Barrett. 1999. High dietary salt enhances acute depressor responses to metformin. *Am J Hypertens* 12(12 Pt 1–2): 1256–1259.

79. Tuck, M. L., et al. 1981. The effect of weight reduction on blood pressure, plasma renin activity, and plasma aldosterone levels in obese patients. *N Engl J Med* 304(16): 930–933.

80. Whitworth, J. A., et al. 1995. Mechanisms of cortisol-induced hypertension in humans. *Steroids* 60(1): 76–80.

81. Bruckdorfer, K. R., et al. 1974. Diurnal changes in the concentrations of plasma lipids, sugars, insulin and corticosterone in rats fed diets containing various carbohydrates. *Horm Metab Res* 6(2): 99–106; Cawley, N. X. 2012. Sugar making sugar: gluconeogenesis triggered by fructose via a hypothalamic-adrenal-corticosterone circuit. *Endocrinology* 153(8): 3561–3563; Kovacevic, S., et al. 2014. Dietary fructose-related adiposity and glucocorticoid receptor function in visceral adipose tissue of female rats. *Eur J Nutr* 53(6): 1409–1420; Bursac, B. N., et al. 2013. Fructose consumption enhances glucocorticoid action in rat visceral adipose tissue. *J Nutr Biochem* 24(6): 1166–1172; London, E., and T. W. Castonguay. High fructose diets increase 11beta-hydroxysteroid dehydrogenase type 1 in liver and visceral adipose in rats within 24-h exposure. *Obesity (Silver Spring)* 19(5): 925–932.

82. Bruckdorfer. Diurnal changes in the concentrations of plasma lipids, sugars, insulin and corticosterone in rats fed diets containing various carbohydrates. 99–106.

83. Perera, G. A. 1950. The adrenal cortex and hypertension. *Bull N Y Acad Med* 26(2): 75–92; Perera, G. A., and D. W. Blood. 1947. The relationship of sodium chloride to hypertension. *J Clin Invest* 26(6): 1109–1118.

84. Cawley. Sugar making sugar: gluconeogenesis triggered by fructose via a hypothalamic-adrenal-corticosterone circuit. 3561–3563.

85. Lanaspa, M. A., et al. 2014. Endogenous fructose production and fructokinase activation mediate renal injury in diabetic nephropathy. *J Am Soc Nephrol* 25(11): 2526–2538; Tang, W. H., K. A. Martin, and J. Hwa. 2012. Aldose reductase, oxidative stress, and diabetic mellitus. *Front Pharmacol* 3: 87.

86. Perera and Blood. The relationship of sodium chloride to hypertension. 1109–1118.

87. Denton, D. 1982. *The Hunger for Salt: An Anthropological, Physiological and Medical Analysis.* New York: Springer-Verlag.

88. McCarty, M. F., and J. J. DiNicolantonio. 2014. Are organically grown foods safer and more healthful than conventionally grown foods? *Br J Nutr* 112(10): 1589–1591.

89. Yamagishi, K., et al. 2010. Dietary intake of saturated fatty acids and mortality from cardiovascular disease in Japanese: the Japan Collaborative Cohort Study for Evaluation of Cancer Risk (JACC) Study. *Am J Clin Nutr* 92(4): 759–765.

90. Sasaki. High blood pressure and the salt intake of the Japanese. 313–324.

91. Timio, M. Blood pressure trend and cardiovascular events in nuns in a secluded order: a 30-year follow-up study. 81–87.

92. Heaney. Making sense of the science of sodium. 63–66; Hollenberg, N. K., et al. 1997. Aging, acculturation, salt intake, and hypertension in the Kuna of Panama. *Hypertension* 29(1 Pt 2): 171–176.

93. Rouse, I. L., B. K. Armstrong, and L. J. Beilin. The relationship of blood pressure to diet and lifestyle in two religious populations. *J Hypertens* 1(1): 65–71.

94. Gleibermann, L. 1973. Blood pressure and dietary salt in human populations. *Ecol Food Nutr* 2(2): 143–156.

95. Ibid.

96. Ibid.

97. Gleibermann. Blood pressure and dietary salt in human populations. 143–156; http://goafrica.about.com/od/Best-Time-to-Visit-Africa/a/Rainy-Seasons-And-Dry-Seasons-In-Africa.htm.

98. Gleibermann. Blood pressure and dietary salt in human populations. 143–156.

99. Kawasaki, T., et al. 1993. Investigation of high salt intake in a Nepalese population with low blood pressure. *J Hum Hypertens* 7(2): 131–140.

100. Gleibermann. Blood pressure and dietary salt in human populations. 143–156.

101. Ibid.

102. Sasaki, N. 1962. High blood pressure and the salt intake of the Japanese. *Jpn Heart J* 3: 313–324.

103. Gleibermann. Blood pressure and dietary salt in human populations. 143–156.

104. Ibid.

105. Swales, J. D. 1980. Dietary salt and hypertension. *Lancet* 1(8179): 1177–1179; Henry, J. P., and J. C. Cassel. Psychosocial factors in essential hypertension. Recent epidemiologic and animal experimental evidence. *Am J Epidemiol* 90(3): 171–200.

106. Sasaki. High blood pressure and the salt intake of the Japanese. 313–324.

107. Iimura, O., et al. 1981. Studies on the hypotensive effect of high potassium intake in patients with essential hypertension. *Clin Sci (Lond)* 61(Suppl 7): 77s–80s.

108. Rouse, Armstrong, and Beilin. The relationship of blood pressure to diet and lifestyle in two religious populations. 65–71.

109. Moore. *The High Blood Pressure Solution.*

110. DiNicolantonio, J. J., S. C. Lucan, and J. H. O'Keefe. 2016. The evidence for saturated fat and for sugar related to coronary heart disease. *Prog Cardiovasc Dis* 58(5): 464–472.

111. http://www.iom.edu/Reports/2013/Sodium-Intake-in-Populations -Assessment-of-Evidence/Report-Brief051413.aspx.

112. Heaney. Making sense of the science of sodium. 63–66.

113. Catanozi, S., et al. 2003. Dietary sodium chloride restriction enhances aortic wall lipid storage and raises plasma lipid concentration in LDL receptor knockout mice. *J Lipid Res* 44(4): 727–732; Ivanovski, O., et al. 2005. Dietary salt restriction accelerates atherosclerosis in apolipoprotein E-deficient mice. *Atherosclerosis* 180(2): 271–276.

114. Nakandakare, E. R., et al. 2008. Dietary salt restriction increases plasma lipoprotein and inflammatory marker concentrations in hypertensive patients. *Atherosclerosis* 200(2): 410–416.

115. Dzau, V. J. 1988. Mechanism of the interaction of hypertension and hypercholesterolemia in atherogenesis: the effects of antihypertensive agents. *Am Heart J* 116(6 Pt 2): 1725–1728; Leren, T. P. 1985. Doxazosin increases low density lipoprotein receptor activity. *Acta Pharmacol Toxicol (Copenh)* 56(3): 269–272.

116. Masugi, F., et al. 1988. Changes in plasma lipids and uric acid with sodium loading and sodium depletion in patients with essential hypertension. *J Hum Hypertens* 1(4): 293–298.

117. Harsha, D. W., et al. 2004. Effect of dietary sodium intake on blood lipids: results from the DASH-sodium trial. *Hypertension* 43(2): 393–398.

118. Krikken, J. A., et al. 2012. Short term dietary sodium restriction decreases HDL cholesterol, apolipoprotein A-I and high molecular weight adiponectin in healthy young men: relationships with renal hemodynamics and RAAS activation. *Nutr Metab Cardiovasc Dis* 22(1): 35–41.

119. Graudal, N. A., T. Hubeck-Graudal, and G. Jurgens. 2011. Effects of low sodium diet versus high sodium diet on blood pressure, renin, aldosterone, catecholamines, cholesterol, and triglyceride. *Cochrane Database Syst Rev* (11): Cd004022.

120. Weder, A. B., and B. M. Egan. 1991. Potential deleterious impact of dietary salt restriction on cardiovascular risk factors. *Klin Wochenschr* 69(Suppl 25): 45–50.

121. Rillaerts, E., et al. 1989. Blood viscosity in human obesity: relation to glucose tolerance and insulin status. *Int J Obes* 13(6): 739–745.

122. Overlack. Divergent hemodynamic and hormonal responses to varying salt intake in normotensive subjects. 331–338; Dimsdale, J. E., et al. 1990. Prediction of salt sensitivity. *Am J Hypertens* 3(6 Pt 1): 429–435.

123. Graudal, Hubeck-Graudal, and Jurgens. Effects of low sodium diet versus high sodium diet on blood pressure, renin, aldosterone, catecholamines, cholesterol, and triglyceride. Cd004022.

124. Weder and Egan. Potential deleterious impact of dietary salt restriction on cardiovascular risk factors. 45–50.

125. Ibid.

126. Alderman, M. H., et al. 1995. Low urinary sodium is associated with greater risk of myocardial infarction among treated hypertensive men. *Hypertension* 25(6): 1144–1152.

127. Stolarz-Skrzypek, K., et al. 2011. Fatal and nonfatal outcomes, incidence of hypertension, and blood pressure changes in relation to urinary sodium excretion. *JAMA* 305(17): 1777–1785.

128. O'Donnell, M., et al. 2014. Urinary sodium and potassium excretion, mortality, and cardiovascular events. *N Engl J Med* 371(7): 612–623.

129. Graudal, N., et al. 2014. Compared with usual sodium intake, low- and excessive-sodium diets are associated with increased mortality: a meta-analysis. *Am J Hypertens* 27(9): 1129–1137.

CHAPTER 5: WE ARE STARVING INSIDE

1. http://www.cdc.gov/nchs/data/hestat/obesity_adult_09_10/obesity_adult_09_10.htm.

2. Lucan, S. C., and J. J. DiNicolantonio. 2015. How calorie-focused thinking about obesity and related diseases may mislead and harm public health. An alternative. *Public Health Nutr* 18(4): 571–581; Bray, G. A., S. J. Nielsen, and B. M. Popkin. 2004. Consumption of high-fructose corn syrup in beverages may play a role in the epidemic of obesity. *Am J Clin Nutr* 79(4): 537–543; DiNicolantonio, J. J. 2014. The cardiometabolic consequences of replacing saturated fats with carbohydrates or Ω-6 polyunsaturated fats: do the dietary guidelines have it wrong? *Open Heart* 1: e000032. doi:10.1136/openhrt-2013-000032.

3. Taubes, G. 2007. *Good Calories, Bad Calories.* New York: Knopf; Prada, P. O., et al. 2005. Low salt intake modulates insulin signaling, JNK activity and IRS-1ser307 phosphorylation in rat tissues. *J Endocrinol* 185(3): 429–437; Garg, R., et al. 2011. Low-salt diet increases insulin resistance in healthy subjects. *Metabolism* 60(7): 965–968.

4. Weidemann, B. J., et al. 2015. Dietary sodium suppresses digestive efficiency via the renin-angiotensin system. *Sci Rep* 5: 11123.

5. Taubes. *Good Calories, Bad Calories.*

6. Gupta, N., K. K. Jani, and N. Gupta. 2011. Hypertension: salt restriction, sodium homeostasis, and other ions. *Indian J Med Sci* 65(3): 121–132.

7. Taubes. *Good Calories, Bad Calories.*

8. Lustig, R. H. 2011. Hypothalamic obesity after craniopharyngioma: mechanisms, diagnosis, and treatment. *Front Endocrinol* 2: 60.

9. Taubes. *Good Calories, Bad Calories.*

10. Prada. Low salt intake modulates insulin signaling, JNK activity and IRS-1ser307 phosphorylation in rat tissues. 429–437; Leandro, S. M., et al. 2008. Low birth weight in response to salt restriction during pregnancy is not due to alterations in uterine-placental blood flow or the placental and peripheral renin-angiotensin system. *Physiol Behav* 95(1–2): 145–151; Lopes, K. L., et al. 2008. Perinatal salt restriction: a new pathway to programming adiposity indices in adult female Wistar rats. *Life Sci* 82(13–14): 728–732; Vidonho, A. F., Jr., et al. 2004. Perinatal salt restriction: a new pathway to programming insulin resistance and dyslipidemia in adult Wistar rats. *Pediatr Res* 56(6): 842–848.

11. Wilcox, G. 2005. Insulin and insulin resistance. *Clin Biochem Rev* 26(2): 19–39; http://www.news-medical.net/health/Insulin-Resistance

-Diagnosis.aspx; Wu, T., et al. 2002. Associations of serum C-reactive protein with fasting insulin, glucose, and glycosylated hemoglobin: the Third National Health and Nutrition Examination Survey, 1988–1994. Am J Epidemiol 155(1): 65–71; Palaniappan, L. P., M. R. Carnethon, and S. P. Fortmann. Heterogeneity in the relationship between ethnicity, BMI, and fasting insulin. Diabetes Care 25(8): 1351–1357; Lindeberg, S., et al. 1999. Low serum insulin in traditional Pacific Islanders—the Kitava Study. Metabolism 48(10): 1216–1219; Lindgarde, F., et al. 2004. Traditional versus agricultural lifestyle among Shuar women of the Ecuadorian Amazon: effects on leptin levels. Metabolism 53(10): 1355–1358.

12. Patel, S. M., et al. 2015. Dietary sodium reduction does not affect circulating glucose concentrations in fasting children or adults: findings from a systematic review and meta-analysis. J Nutr 145(3): 505–513.

13. Egan, B. M., K. Stepniakowski, and P. Nazzaro. 1994. Insulin levels are similar in obese salt-sensitive and salt-resistant hypertensive subjects. Hypertension 23(1 Suppl): I1–I7; Egan, B. M., and K. Stepniakowski. 1993. Effects of enalapril on the hyperinsulinemic response to severe salt restriction in obese young men with mild systemic hypertension. Am J Cardiol 72(1): 53–57; Egan, B. M., and K. T. Stepniakowski. 1997. Adverse effects of short-term, very-low-salt diets in subjects with risk-factor clustering. Am J Clin Nutr 65(2 Suppl): 671s–677s.

14. Iwaoka, T., et al. 1988. The effect of low and high NaCl diets on oral glucose tolerance. Klin Wochenschr 66(16): 724–728.

15. Egan, B. M., K. Stepniakowski, and T. L. Goodfriend. 1994. Renin and aldosterone are higher and the hyperinsulinemic effect of salt restriction greater in subjects with risk factors clustering. Am J Hypertens 7(10 Pt 1): 886–893.

16. Egan and Stepniakowski. Adverse effects of short-term, very-low-salt diets in subjects with risk-factor clustering. 671s–677s.

17. Ibid.

18. Egan, B. M., and D. T. Lackland. 2000. Biochemical and metabolic effects of very-low-salt diets. Am J Med Sci 320(4): 233–239.

19. Ruppert, M., et al. 1991. Short-term dietary sodium restriction increases serum lipids and insulin in salt-sensitive and salt-resistant normotensive adults. Klin Wochenschr 69(Suppl 25): 51–57.

20. Patel. Dietary sodium reduction does not affect circulating glucose concentrations in fasting children or adults: findings from a systematic review and meta-analysis. 505–513; Egan, Stepniakowski, and Nazzaro. Insulin levels are similar in obese salt-sensitive and salt-resistant hypertensive subjects. I1–I7; Egan and Stepniakowski. Effects of enal-

april on the hyperinsulinemic response to severe salt restriction in obese young men with mild systemic hypertension. 53–57.

21. Egan, B. M., et al. 1991. Neurohumoral and metabolic effects of short-term dietary NaCl restriction in men. Relationship to salt-sensitivity status. *Am J Hypertens* 4(5 Pt 1): 416–421.

22. Prada, P., et al. 2000. High- or low-salt diet from weaning to adulthood: effect on insulin sensitivity in Wistar rats. *Hypertension* 35(1 Pt 2): 424–429.

23. Okamoto, M. M., et al. 2004. Changes in dietary sodium consumption modulate GLUT4 gene expression and early steps of insulin signaling. *Am J Physiol Regul Integr Comp Physiol* 286(4): R779–R785.

24. Iwaoka. The effect of low and high NaCl diets on oral glucose tolerance. 724–728; Ruppert. Short-term dietary sodium restriction increases serum lipids and insulin in salt-sensitive and salt-resistant normotensive adults. 51–57; Sharma, A. M., et al. 1990. Dietary sodium restriction: adverse effect on plasma lipids. *Klin Wochenschr* 68(13): 664–668.

25. Prada. High- or low-salt diet from weaning to adulthood: effect on insulin sensitivity in Wistar rats. 424–429.

26. Xavier, A. R., et al. 2003. Dietary sodium restriction exacerbates age-related changes in rat adipose tissue and liver lipogenesis. *Metabolism* 52(8): 1072–1077.

27. Ames, R. P. 2001. The effect of sodium supplementation on glucose tolerance and insulin concentrations in patients with hypertension and diabetes mellitus. *Am J Hypertens* 14(7 Pt 1): 653–659.

28. McCarty, M. F. 2004. Elevated sympathetic activity may promote insulin resistance syndrome by activating alpha-1 adrenergic receptors on adipocytes. *Med Hypotheses* 62(5): 830–838.

29. Ibid; Pollare, T., H. Lithell, and C. Berne. 1989. A comparison of the effects of hydrochlorothiazide and captopril on glucose and lipid metabolism in patients with hypertension. *N Engl J Med* 321(13): 868–873.

30. DiNicolantonio, J. J., J. H. O'Keefe, and S. C. Lucan. Added fructose: a principal driver of type 2 diabetes mellitus and its consequences. *Mayo Clin Proc* 90(3): 372–381.

31. Lustig, R. H. 2010. Fructose: metabolic, hedonic, and societal parallels with ethanol. *J Am Diet Assoc* 110(9): 1307–1321.

32. Bursac, B. N., et al. 2014. High-fructose diet leads to visceral adiposity and hypothalamic leptin resistance in male rats—do glucocorticoids play a role? *J Nutr Biochem* 25(4): 446–455.

33. Lim, J. S., et al. 2010. The role of fructose in the pathogenesis of NAFLD and the metabolic syndrome. *Nat Rev Gastroenterol Hepatol* 7(5): 251–264; Abdelmalek, M. F., et al. 2012. Higher dietary fructose is associated with impaired hepatic adenosine triphosphate homeostasis in obese individuals with type 2 diabetes. *Hepatology* 56(3): 952–960.

34. Palmer, B. F., and D. J. Clegg. 2015. Electrolyte and acid-base disturbances in patients with diabetes mellitus. *N Engl J Med* 373(6): 548–559.

CHAPTER 6: CRYSTAL REHAB: USING SALT CRAVINGS TO KICK SUGAR ADDICTION

1. https://books.google.com/books?id=WuMRAAAAYAAJ&pg= PA364&dq=Lapicque+salt&hl=en&sa=X&ved=0ahUKEwj9uc SG6bnPAhWJ8z4KHd-3BLAQ6AEIKDAC#v=onepage&q= Lapicque&f=false.

2. https://books.google.com/books?id=NIdYAAAAMAAJ&pg= PA441&lpg=PA441&dq=m.+lapicque+salt&source=bl&ots= KOUJakgy-A&sig=4QvDiiNRHZ3xXEonXtoZUo4VH_8&hl=en &sa=X&ved=0ahUKEwjMgZvu6bnPAhXLOD4KHaILCbEQ6A EIHDAA#v=onepage&q=m.%20lapicque%20salt&f=false.

3. Dorhout Mees, E. J., and T. Thien. 2008. Beyond science: the salt debate. *Neth J Med* 66(10): 404–407.

4. Meneely, G. R., and H. D. Battarbee. 1976. High sodium-low potassium environment and hypertension. *Am J Cardiol* 38(6): 768–785.

5. Ibid.

6. Ghooi, R. B., V. V. Valanju, and M. G. Rajarshi. 1993. Salt restriction in hypertension. *Med Hypotheses* 41(2): 137–140.

7. Denton, D. 1982. *The Hunger for Salt: An Anthropological, Physiological and Medical Analysis.* New York: Springer-Verlag; Ghooi, Valanju, and Rajarshi. Salt restriction in hypertension. 137–140.

8. Folkow, B. 2003. [Salt and blood pressure—centenarian bone of contention]. *Lakartidningen* 100(40): 3142–3147. [Article in Swedish]; Wald, N., and M. Leshem. 2003. Salt conditions a flavor preference or aversion after exercise depending on NaCl dose and sweat loss. *Appetite* 40(3): 277–284; Leshem, M., A. Abutbul, and R. Eilon. 1999. Exercise increases the preference for salt in humans. *Appetite* 32(2): 251–260; Leshem, M., and J. Rudoy. 1997. Hemodialysis increases the preference for salt in soup. *Physiol Behav* 61(1): 65–69.

9. DiNicolantonio, J. J., and S. C. Lucan. 2014. The wrong white crystals: not salt but sugar as aetiological in hypertension and cardiometabolic disease. *Open Heart* 1. doi:10.1136/openhrt-2014-000167.

10. Folkow. [Salt and blood pressure—centenarian bone of contention].
    3142–3147.

11. Titze, J., et al. 2016. Balancing wobbles in the body sodium. *Nephrol
    Dial Transplant* 31(7): 1078–1081.

12. Dahl, L. K. 2005. Possible role of salt intake in the development of es-
    sential hypertension. 1960. *Int J Epidemiol* 34(5): 967–972; discussion
    972–974, 975–978.

13. Wassertheil-Smoller, S., et al. 1992. The Trial of Antihypertensive
    Interventions and Management (TAIM) Study. Final results with re-
    gard to blood pressure, cardiovascular risk, and quality of life. *Am J
    Hypertens* 5(1): 37–44.

14. Heaney, R. P. 2015. Making sense of the science of sodium. *Nutr Today*
    50(2): 63–66.

15. Clark, J. J., and I. L. Bernstein. 2006. A role for D2 but not D1 dopa-
    mine receptors in the cross-sensitization between amphetamine and
    salt appetite. *Pharmacol Biochem Behav* 83(2): 277–284; Robinson,
    T. E., and K. C. Berridge 1993. The neural basis of drug craving: an
    incentive-sensitization theory of addiction. *Brain Res Rev* 18(3): 247–
    291; McCutcheon, B., and C. Levy. 1972. Relationship between NaCl
    rewarded bar-pressing and duration of sodium deficiency. *Physiol Behav*
    8(4): 761–763.

16. Sakai, R. R., et al. 1987. Salt appetite is enhanced by one prior episode
    of sodium depletion in the rat. *Behav Neurosci* 101(5): 724–731.

17. Denton, D. A., M. J. McKinley, and R. S. Weisinger. 1996. Hypotha-
    lamic integration of body fluid regulation. *Proc Natl Acad Sci U S A*
    93(14): 7397–7404; Liedtke, W. B., et al. 2011. Relation of addiction
    genes to hypothalamic gene changes subserving genesis and gratifica-
    tion of a classic instinct, sodium appetite. *Proc Natl Acad Sci U S A*
    108(30): 12509–12514.

18. Robinson and Berridge. The neural basis of drug craving: an incentive-
    sensitization theory of addiction. 247–291.

19. Clark and Bernstein. A role for D2 but not D1 dopamine receptors in
    the cross-sensitization between amphetamine and salt appetite. 277–
    284; Roitman, M. F., et al. 2002. Induction of a salt appetite alters
    dendritic morphology in nucleus accumbens and sensitizes rats to am-
    phetamine. *J Neurosci* 22(11): Rc225; Robinson, T. E., and B. Kolb.
    1997. Persistent structural modifications in nucleus accumbens and
    prefrontal cortex neurons produced by previous experience with am-
    phetamine. *J Neurosci* 17(21): 8491–8497.

20. Clark, J. J., and I. L. Bernstein 2004. Reciprocal cross-sensitization
    between amphetamine and salt appetite. *Pharmacol Biochem Behav*

78(4): 691–698; Vanderschuren, L. J., et al. 1999. Dopaminergic mechanisms mediating the long-term expression of locomotor sensitization following pre-exposure to morphine or amphetamine. *Psychopharmacology (Berl)* 143(3): 244–253.

21. Vanderschuren. Dopaminergic mechanisms mediating the long-term expression of locomotor sensitization following pre-exposure to morphine or amphetamine. 244–253.

22. Cocores, J. A., and M. S. Gold. 2009. The Salted Food Addiction Hypothesis may explain overeating and the obesity epidemic. *Med Hypotheses* 73(6): 892–899.

23. Heaney. Making sense of the science of sodium. 63–66; Wald and Leshem. Salt conditions a flavor preference or aversion after exercise depending on NaCl dose and sweat loss. 277–284.

24. Heaney. Making sense of the science of sodium. 63–66.

25. http://www.drugabuse.gov/related-topics/trends-statistics/overdose-death-rates.

26. Fessler, D. M. 2003. An evolutionary explanation of the plasticity of salt preferences: prophylaxis against sudden dehydration. *Med Hypotheses* 61(3): 412–415.

27. Ibid.

28. Shirazki, A., et al. 2007. Lowest neonatal serum sodium predicts sodium intake in low birth weight children. *Am J Physiol Regul Integr Comp Physiol* 292(4): R1683–R1689.

29. Leshem, M. 2011. Low dietary sodium is anxiogenic in rats. *Physiol Behav* 103(5): 453–458.

30. http://www.medicalnewstoday.com/releases/141778.php.

31. Pines, K. L., and G. A. Perera. 1949. Sodium chloride restriction in hypertensive vascular disease. *Med Clin North Am* 33(3): 713–725.

32. Tryon, M. S., et al. Excessive sugar consumption may be a difficult habit to break: a view from the brain and body. *J Clin Endocrinol Metab* 100(6): 2239–2247; Tryon, M. S., et al. 2013. Chronic stress exposure may affect the brain's response to high calorie food cues and predispose to obesogenic eating habits. *Physiol Behav* 120: 233–242.

33. Yudkin, J. 2012. *Pure, white and deadly: how sugar is killing us and what we can do to stop it*. New York: Penguin.

34. DiNicolantonio, J. J., and S. C. Lucan. 2014. Sugar season: it's everywhere and addictive. *New York Times*, December 12.

35. Ibid.

36. Newhauser, R. 2013. John Gower's sweet tooth. *Rev Engl Stud* 64(267): 752–769.

37. DiNicolantonio, J. J., J. H. O'Keefe, and S. C. Lucan, Added fructose: a principal driver of type 2 diabetes mellitus and its consequences. *Mayo Clin Proc* 90(3): 372–381.

38. Ahmed, S. H., K. Guillem, and Y. Vandaele. 2013. Sugar addiction: pushing the drug-sugar analogy to the limit. *Curr Opin Clin Nutr Metab Care* 16(4): 434–439.

39. DiNicolantonio and Lucan. Sugar season: it's everywhere and addictive.

40. Avena, N. M., P. Rada, and B. G. Hoebel. 2008. Evidence for sugar addiction: behavioral and neurochemical effects of intermittent, excessive sugar intake. *Neurosci Biobehav Rev* 32(1): 20–39; Colantuoni, C., et al. 2002. Evidence that intermittent, excessive sugar intake causes endogenous opioid dependence. *Obes Res* 10(6): 478–488; Colantuoni, C., et al. 2001. Excessive sugar intake alters binding to dopamine and mu-opioid receptors in the brain. *Neuroreport* 12(16): 3549–3552; Unterwald, E. M., J. Fillmore, and M. J. Kreek. 1996. Chronic repeated cocaine administration increases dopamine D1 receptor-mediated signal transduction. *Eur J Pharmacol* 318(1): 31–35; Vanderschuren, L. J., and P. W. Kalivas. 2000. Alterations in dopaminergic and glutamatergic transmission in the induction and expression of behavioral sensitization: a critical review of preclinical studies. *Psychopharmacology (Berl)* 151(2–3): 99–120.

41. Bray, G. A., S. J. Nielsen, and B. M. Popkin. 2004. Consumption of high-fructose corn syrup in beverages may play a role in the epidemic of obesity. *Am J Clin Nutr* 79(4): 537–543; Bursac, B. N., et al. 2014. High-fructose diet leads to visceral adiposity and hypothalamic leptin resistance in male rats—do glucocorticoids play a role? *J Nutr Biochem* 25(4): 446–455; Shapiro, A., et al. 2008. Fructose-induced leptin resistance exacerbates weight gain in response to subsequent high-fat feeding. *Am J Physiol Regul Integr Comp Physiol* 295(5): R1370–R1375; Shapiro, A., et al. 2011. Prevention and reversal of diet-induced leptin resistance with a sugar-free diet despite high fat content. *Br J Nutr* 106(3): 390–397.

42. Taubes, G. 2007. *Good Calories, Bad Calories*. New York: Knopf.

43. DiNicolantonio and Lucan. Sugar season: it's everywhere and addictive.

CHAPTER 7: HOW MUCH SALT DO YOU REALLY NEED?

1. Simpson, F. O. 1990. The control of body sodium in relation to hypertension: exploring the Strauss concept. *J Cardiovasc Pharmacol* 16(Suppl 7): S27–S30.

2. Hollenberg, N. K. 1980. Set point for sodium homeostasis: surfeit, deficit, and their implications. *Kidney Int* 17(4): 423–429.

3. Andrukhova, O., et al. 2014. FGF23 regulates renal sodium handling and blood pressure. *EMBO Mol Med* 6(6): 744–759.

4. Hollenberg. Set point for sodium homeostasis: surfeit, deficit, and their implications. 423–429.

5. Ibid.

6. Strauss, M. B., et al. 1958. Surfeit and deficit of sodium: a kinetic concept of sodium excretion. *AMA Arch Intern Med* 102(4): 527–536.

7. https://en.wikipedia.org/wiki/Intravascular_volume_status.

8. Peters, J. P. 1950. Sodium, water and edema. *J Mt Sinai Hosp N Y* 17(3): 159–175.

9. Gupta, N., K. K. Jani, and N. Gupta. 2011. Hypertension: salt restriction, sodium homeostasis, and other ions. *Indian J Med Sci* 65(3): 121–132.

10. Elkinton, J. R., T. S. Danowski, and A. W. Winkler. 1946. Hemodynamic changes in salt depletion and in dehydration. *J Clin Invest* 25: 120–129.

11. Ibid.

12. Gankam-Kengne, F., et al. 2013. Mild hyponatremia is associated with an increased risk of death in an ambulatory setting. *Kidney Int* 83(4): 700–706.

13. AlZahrani, A., R. Sinnert, and J. Gernsheimer. 2013. Acute kidney injury, sodium disorders, and hypercalcemia in the aging kidney: diagnostic and therapeutic management strategies in emergency medicine. *Clin Geriatr Med* 29(1): 275–319.

14. Kovesdy, C. P., et al. 2012. Hyponatremia, hypernatremia, and mortality in patients with chronic kidney disease with and without congestive heart failure. *Circulation* 125(5): 677–684; Delin, K., et al. 1984. Factors regulating sodium balance in proctocolectomized patients with various ileal resections. *Scand J Gastroenterol* 19(2): 145–149.

15. Passare, G., et al. 2004. Sodium and potassium disturbances in the elderly: prevalence and association with drug use. *Clin Drug Investig* 24(9): 535–544.

16. Kovesdy. Hyponatremia, hypernatremia, and mortality in patients with chronic kidney disease with and without congestive heart failure. 677–684.

17. Wannamethee, S. G., et al. 2016. Mild hyponatremia, hypernatremia and incident cardiovascular disease and mortality in older men:

a population-based cohort study. *Nutr Metab Cardiovasc Dis* 26(1): 12–19.

18. AlZahrani, Sinnert, and Gernsheimer. Acute kidney injury, sodium disorders, and hypercalcemia in the aging kidney: diagnostic and therapeutic management strategies in emergency medicine. 275–319.

19. Kovesdy, C. P. 2012. Significance of hypo- and hypernatremia in chronic kidney disease. *Nephrol Dial Transplant* 27(3): 891–898.

20. AlZahrani, Sinnert, and Gernsheimer. Acute kidney injury, sodium disorders, and hypercalcemia in the aging kidney: diagnostic and therapeutic management strategies in emergency medicine. 275–319.

21. Bautista, A. A., J. E. Duya, and M. A. Sandoval. 2014. Salt-losing nephropathy in hypothyroidism. *BMJ Case Rep.* doi:10.1136/bcr-2014-203895.

22. Schoenfeld, P. 2013. Safety of MiraLAX/Gatorade bowel preparation has not been established in appropriately designed studies. *Clin Gastroenterol Hepatol* 11(5): 582.

23. Cohen, L. B., D. M. Kastenberg, D. B. Mount, and A. V. Safdi. 2009. Current issues in optimal bowel preparation: excerpts from a round-table discussion among colon-cleansing experts. *Gastroenterol Hepatol (N Y)* 5(11 Suppl 19): 3–11.

24. Wolfe, M. M., D. R. Lichtenstein, and G. Singh. 1999. Gastrointestinal toxicity of nonsteroidal antiinflammatory drugs. *N Engl J Med* 340(24): 1888–1899.

25. Sharp, R. L. 2006. Role of sodium in fluid homeostasis with exercise. *J Am Coll Nutr* 25(3 Suppl): 231s–239s.

26. Ghooi, R. B., V. V. Valanju, and M. G. Rajarshi. 1993. Salt restriction in hypertension. *Med Hypotheses* 41(2): 137–140.

27. Mao, I. F., M. L. Chen, and Y. C. Ko. 2001. Electrolyte loss in sweat and iodine deficiency in a hot environment. *Arch Environ Health* 56(3): 271–277.

28. Ghooi, Valanju, and Rajarshi. Salt restriction in hypertension. 137–140; Mao, Chen, and Ko. Electrolyte loss in sweat and iodine deficiency in a hot environment. 271–277.

29. Mao, Chen, and Ko. Electrolyte loss in sweat and iodine deficiency in a hot environment. 271–277.

30. Blank, M. C., et al. 2012. Total body Na(+)-depletion without hyponatraemia can trigger overtraining-like symptoms with sleeping disorders and increasing blood pressure: explorative case and literature study. *Med Hypotheses* 79(6): 799–804.

31. Noakes, T. 2002. Hyponatremia in distance runners: fluid and sodium balance during exercise. *Curr Sports Med Rep* 1(4): 197–207.

32. Mao, Chen, and Ko. Electrolyte loss in sweat and iodine deficiency in a hot environment. 271–277.

33. Blank. Total body Na(+)-depletion without hyponatraemia can trigger overtraining-like symptoms with sleeping disorders and increasing blood pressure: explorative case and literature study. 799–804.

34. Ibid; Shirreffs, S. M., et al. 1996. Post-exercise rehydration in man: effects of volume consumed and drink sodium content. *Med Sci Sports Exerc* 28(10): 1260–1271.

35. Sharp. Role of sodium in fluid homeostasis with exercise. 231s–239s.

36. Blank. Total body Na(+)-depletion without hyponatraemia can trigger overtraining-like symptoms with sleeping disorders and increasing blood pressure: explorative case and literature study. 799–804.

37. Sharp. Role of sodium in fluid homeostasis with exercise. 231s–239s.

38. Sanders, B., T. D. Noakes, and S. C. Dennis. 2001. Sodium replacement and fluid shifts during prolonged exercise in humans. *Eur J Appl Physiol* 84(5): 419–425.

39. Sharp. Role of sodium in fluid homeostasis with exercise. 231s–239s.

40. Sutters, M., R. Duncan, and W. S. Peart. 1995. Effect of dietary salt restriction on renal sensitivity to vasopressin in man. *Clin Sci (Lond)* 89(1): 37–43.

41. Moinier, B. M., and T. B. Drueke. 2008. Aphrodite, sex and salt—from butterfly to man. *Nephrol Dial Transplant* 23(7): 2154–2161.

42. Wassertheil-Smoller, S., et al. 1991. Effect of antihypertensives on sexual function and quality of life: the TAIM Study. *Ann Intern Med* 114(8): 613–620.

43. Jaaskelainen, J., A. Tiitinen, and R. Voutilainen. 2001. Sexual function and fertility in adult females and males with congenital adrenal hyperplasia. *Horm Res* 56(3–4): 73–80.

44. Osteria, T. S. 1982. Maternal nutrition, infant health, and subsequent fertility. *Philipp J Nutr* 35(3): 106–111.

45. Leandro, S. M., et al. 2008. Low birth weight in response to salt restriction during pregnancy is not due to alterations in uterine-placental blood flow or the placental and peripheral renin-angiotensin system. *Physiol Behav* 95(1–2): 145–151; Lopes, K. L., et al. 2008. Perinatal salt restriction: a new pathway to programming adiposity indices in adult female Wistar rats. *Life Sci* 82(13–14): 728–732; Vidonho, A. F., Jr., et al. 2004. Perinatal salt restriction: a new pathway to programming

insulin resistance and dyslipidemia in adult Wistar rats. *Pediatr Res* 56(6): 842–848.

46. Battista, M. C., et al. 2002. Intrauterine growth restriction in rats is associated with hypertension and renal dysfunction in adulthood. *Am J Physiol Endocrinol Metab* 283(1): E124–E131.

47. http://www.who.int/nutrition/publications/guidelines/sodium _intake_printversion.pdf.

48. Zimmermann, M. B. 2012. The effects of iodine deficiency in pregnancy and infancy. *Paediatr Perinat Epidemiol* 26(Suppl 1): 108–117.

49. http://www.who.int/nutrition/publications/micronutrients /PHN10(12a).pdf.

50. Campbell, N. R., et al. 2012. Need for coordinated programs to improve global health by optimizing salt and iodine intake. *Rev Panam Salud Publica* 32(4): 281–286.

51. Zimmermann, M. B. 2012. Are weaning infants at risk of iodine deficiency even in countries with established iodized salt programs? *Nestle Nutr Inst Workshop Ser* 70: 137–146.

52. Jaiswal, N., et al. 2014. High prevalence of maternal hypothyroidism despite adequate iodine status in Indian pregnant women in the first trimester. *Thyroid* 24(9): 1419–1429.

53. Pearce, E. N., M. Andersson, and M. B. Zimmermann. 2013. Global iodine nutrition: where do we stand in 2013? *Thyroid* 23(5): 523–528; Zimmermann, M. B. 2013. Iodine deficiency and excess in children: worldwide status in 2013. *Endocr Pract* 19(5): 839–846.

54. http://www.thyroid.org/crn-releases-science-based-guidelines-on -iodine-in-multivitaminmineral-supplements-for-pregnancy-and -lactation/.

55. Robinson, M. 1958. Salt in pregnancy. *Lancet* 1(7013): 178–181.

56. Ibid.

57. Ibid.

58. Ibid.

59. Duley, L., and D. Henderson-Smart. 2000. Reduced salt intake compared to normal dietary salt, or high intake, in pregnancy. *Cochrane Database Syst Rev* (2): Cd001687.

60. Farese, S., et al. 2006. Blood pressure reduction in pregnancy by sodium chloride. *Nephrol Dial Transplant* 21(7): 1984–1987.

61. Gennari-Moser, C., et al. 2014. Normotensive blood pressure in pregnancy: the role of salt and aldosterone. *Hypertension* 63(2): 362–368.

62. Scholten, R. R., et al. 2015. Low plasma volume in normotensive formerly preeclamptic women predisposes to hypertension. *Hypertension* 66(5): 1066–1072.

63. Farese. Blood pressure reduction in pregnancy by sodium chloride. 1984–1987; Silver, H. M., M. Seebeck, and R. Carlson. 1998. Comparison of total blood volume in normal, preeclamptic, and nonproteinuric gestational hypertensive pregnancy by simultaneous measurement of red blood cell and plasma volumes. *Am J Obstet Gynecol* 179(1): 87–93.

64. Wassertheil-Smoller. Effect of antihypertensives on sexual function and quality of life: the TAIM Study. 613–620.

65. Wassertheil-Smoller, S., et al. 1992. The Trial of Antihypertensive Interventions and Management (TAIM) Study. Final results with regard to blood pressure, cardiovascular risk, and quality of life. *Am J Hypertens* 5(1): 37–44.

66. Ghooi, Valanju, and Rajarshi. Salt restriction in hypertension. 137–140.

67. Wassertheil-Smoller. Effect of antihypertensives on sexual function and quality of life: the TAIM Study. 613–620.

68. Graham, K. F. 2011. Dietary salt restriction and chronic fatigue syndrome: a hypothesis. *Med Hypotheses* 77(3): 462–463; Bou-Holaigah, I., et al. 1995. The relationship between neurally mediated hypotension and the chronic fatigue syndrome. *JAMA* 274(12): 961–967.

69. Feldman, R. D., A. G. Logan, and N. D. Schmidt. 1996. Dietary salt restriction increases vascular insulin resistance. *Clin Pharmacol Ther* 60(4): 444–451; Feldman, R. D., and N. D. Schmidt. 1999. Moderate dietary salt restriction increases vascular and systemic insulin resistance. *Am J Hypertens* 12(6): 643–647.

70. Hollingsworth, K. G., et al. 2010. Impaired cardiovascular response to standing in chronic fatigue syndrome. *Eur J Clin Invest* 40(7): 608–615; Kaiserova, M., et al. 2015. Orthostatic hypotension is associated with decreased cerebrospinal fluid levels of chromogranin A in early stage of Parkinson disease. *Clin Auton Res* 25(5): 339–342.

71. Liamis, G., E. Liberopoulos, F. Barkas, and M. Elisaf. 2014. Diabetes mellitus and electrolyte disorders. *World J Clin Cases* 2(10): 488–496.

72. Palmer, B. F., and D. J. Clegg. 2015. Electrolyte and acid-base disturbances in patients with diabetes mellitus. *N Engl J Med* 373(6): 548–559; Peters. Sodium, water and edema. 159–175; Liamis, Liberopoulos, Barkas, and Elisaf. Diabetes mellitus and electrolyte disorders. 488–496.

73. Ames, R. P. 2001. The effect of sodium supplementation on glucose tolerance and insulin concentrations in patients with hypertension and diabetes mellitus. *Am J Hypertens* 14(7 Pt 1): 653–659.

74. Menke, A., et al. 2015. Prevalence of and trends in diabetes among adults in the United States, 1988–2012. *JAMA* 314(10): 1021–1029.

75. Johnson, R. J. 2012. *The Fat Switch.* Mercola.com.

76. DiNicolantonio, J. J., and S. C. Lucan. 2015. Is fructose malabsorption a cause of irritable bowel syndrome? *Med Hypotheses* 85(3): 295–297.

77. Santelmann, H., and J. M. Howard. 2005. Yeast metabolic products, yeast antigens and yeasts as possible triggers for irritable bowel syndrome. *Eur J Gastroenterol Hepatol* 17(1): 21–26; Buu, L. M., and Y. C. Chen. 2014. Impact of glucose levels on expression of hypha-associated secreted aspartyl proteinases in *Candida albicans. J Biomed Sci* 21: 22; Vargas, S. L., et al. 1993. Modulating effect of dietary carbohydrate supplementation on *Candida albicans* colonization and invasion in a neutropenic mouse model. *Infect Immun* 61(2): 619–626.

78. Nakayama, T., et al. 2010. Dietary fructose causes tubulointerstitial injury in the normal rat kidney. *Am J Physiol Renal Physiol* 298(3): F712–F720.

79. Lanaspa, M. A., et al. 2014. Endogenous fructose production and fructokinase activation mediate renal injury in diabetic nephropathy. *J Am Soc Nephrol* 25(11): 2526–2538.

80. Takeda, R., et al. 1982. [Hyporeninemic hypoaldosteronism associated with diabetes mellitus]. *Nihon Rinsho* 40(9): 2048–2053. [Article in Japanese.]

81. McFarlane, S. I., and J. R. Sowers. 2003. Cardiovascular endocrinology 1: aldosterone function in diabetes mellitus: effects on cardiovascular and renal disease. *J Clin Endocrinol Metab* 88(2): 516–523; Sowers, J. R., and M. Epstein. 1995. Diabetes mellitus and associated hypertension, vascular disease, and nephropathy. An update. *Hypertension* 26(6 Pt 1): 869–879.

82. Sharma, N., et al. High-sugar diets increase cardiac dysfunction and mortality in hypertension compared to low-carbohydrate or high-starch diets. *J Hypertens* 26(7): 1402–1410.

83. Lim, J. S., et al. 2010. The role of fructose in the pathogenesis of NAFLD and the metabolic syndrome. *Nat Rev Gastroenterol Hepatol* 7(5): 251–264.

84. Liamis, Liberopoulos, Barkas, and Elisaf. Diabetes mellitus and electrolyte disorders. 488–496.

85. Ibid.

86. Hillier, T. A., R. D. Abbott, and E. J. Barrett. 1999. Hyponatremia: evaluating the correction factor for hyperglycemia. *Am J Med* 106(4): 399–403.

87. Wannamethee. Mild hyponatremia, hypernatremia and incident cardiovascular disease and mortality in older men: a population-based cohort study. 12–19.

88. Liamis, Liberopoulos, Barkas, and Elisaf. Diabetes mellitus and electrolyte disorders. 488–496.

89. AlZahrani, Sinnert, and Gernsheimer. Acute kidney injury, sodium disorders, and hypercalcemia in the aging kidney: diagnostic and therapeutic management strategies in emergency medicine. 275–319.

90. Liamis, Liberopoulos, Barkas, and Elisaf. Diabetes mellitus and electrolyte disorders. 488–496.

91. AlZahrani, Sinnert, and Gernsheimer. Acute kidney injury, sodium disorders, and hypercalcemia in the aging kidney: diagnostic and therapeutic management strategies in emergency medicine. 275–319; Sachs, J., and B. Fredman. 2006. The hyponatramia of multiple myeloma is true and not pseudohyponatramia. *Med Hypotheses* 67(4): 839–840.

92. Luft, F. C. 2015. Clinical salt deficits. *Pflugers Arch* 467(3): 559–563.

93. Bueter, M., et al. 2011. Sodium and water handling after gastric bypass surgery in a rat model. *Surg Obes Relat Dis* 7(1): 68–73.

94. Bautista, Duya, and Sandoval. Salt-losing nephropathy in hypothyroidism. doi:10.1136/bcr-2014-203895; Vojdani, A., et al. 1996. Immunological cross reactivity between *Candida albicans* and human tissue. *J Clin Lab Immunol* 48(1): 1–15; Santelmann, H. 2007. [A new syndrome?] *Tidsskr Nor Laegeforen* 127(4): 461. [Article in Norwegian.]

95. Bishop, R. F., and G. L. Barnes. 1974. Depression of lactase activity in the small intestine of infant rabbits by *Candida albicans*. *J Med Microbiol* 7(2): 259–263.

96. Santelmann. [A new syndrome?] 461.

97. Ibid; Nieuwenhuizen, W. F., et al. 2003. Is *Candida albicans* a trigger in the onset of coeliac disease? 361(9375): 2152–2154.

98. Agarwal, M., et al. 1999. Hyponatremic-hypertensive syndrome with renal ischemia: an underrecognized disorder. *Hypertension* 33(4): 1020–1024.

99. AlZahrani, Sinnert, and Gernsheimer. Acute kidney injury, sodium disorders, and hypercalcemia in the aging kidney: diagnostic and therapeutic management strategies in emergency medicine. 275–319.

100. Walker, W. G., et al. 1965. Metabolic observations on salt wasting in a patient with renal disease. *Am J Med* 39: 505–519.

101. Faull, C. M., C. Holmes, and P. H. Baylis. Water balance in elderly people: is there a deficiency of vasopressin? *Age Ageing* 22(2): 114–120.

102. Ibid.

103. Scialla, J. J., and C. A. Anderson. 2013. Dietary acid load: a novel nutritional target in chronic kidney disease? *Adv Chronic Kidney Dis* 20(2): 141–149.

104. Faull, Holmes, and Baylis. Water balance in elderly people: is there a deficiency of vasopressin? 114–120; Al-Awqati, Q. 2013. Basic research: Salt wasting in distal renal tubular acidosis—new look, old problem. *Nat Rev Nephrol* 9(12): 712–713.

105. Pines, K. L., and G. A. Perera. 1949. Sodium chloride restriction in hypertensive vascular disease. *Med Clin North Am* 33(3): 713–725; Peters, J. P., et al. 1929. Total acid-base equilibrium of plasma in health and disease: X. The acidosis of nephritis. *J Clin Invest* 6(4): 517–549.

106. Pines and Perera. Sodium chloride restriction in hypertensive vascular disease. 713–725; Mac, G. W., Jr. 1948. Risk of uremia due to sodium depletion. *JAMA* 137(16): 1377; Grollman, A. R., et al. 1945. Sodium restriction in the diet for hypertension. *JAMA* 129(8): 533–537.

107. Schroeder, H. A., et al. 1949. Low sodium chloride diets in hypertension: effects on blood pressure. *JAMA* 140(5): 458–463.

108. Grollman, A. R., et al. 1945. Sodium restriction in the diet for hypertension. *JAMA* 129(8): 533–537.

109. Pines and Perera. Sodium chloride restriction in hypertensive vascular disease. 713–725; Grollman, A. R., et al. 1945. Sodium restriction in the diet for hypertension. *JAMA* 129(8): 533–537.

110. Pines and Perera. Sodium chloride restriction in hypertensive vascular disease. 713–725.

111. Ibid.

112. Kovesdy. Significance of hypo- and hypernatremia in chronic kidney disease. 891–898.

113. Morita, H., et al. 1995. Role of hepatic receptors in controlling body fluid homeostasis. *Jpn J Physiol* 45(3): 355–368; Morita, H., et al. 1993. Hepatorenal reflex plays an important role in natriuresis after high-NaCl food intake in conscious dogs. *Circ Res* 72(3): 552–559; Morita, H., et al. 1990. Effects of portal infusion of hypertonic

solution on jejunal electrolyte transport in anesthetized dogs. *Am J Physiol* 259(6 Pt 2): R1289–R1294; Thomas, L., and R. Kumar 2008. Control of renal solute excretion by enteric signals and mediators. *J Am Soc Nephrol* 19(2): 207–212.

114. Hofmeister, L. H., S. Perisic, and J. Titze. 2015. Tissue sodium storage: evidence for kidney-like extrarenal countercurrent systems? *Pflugers Arch* 467(3): 551–558; Maril, N., et al. 2006. Sodium MRI of the human kidney at 3 Tesla. *Magn Reson Med* 56(6): 1229–1234; Haneder, S., et al. 2011. Quantitative and qualitative (23)Na MR imaging of the human kidneys at 3 T: before and after a water load. *Radiology* 260(3): 857–865.

115. Kovesdy. Significance of hypo- and hypernatremia in chronic kidney disease. 891–898.

116. Ibid.

117. Ibid.

118. Wannamethee. Mild hyponatremia, hypernatremia and incident cardiovascular disease and mortality in older men: a population-based cohort study. 12–19.

119. Kovesdy. Hyponatremia, hypernatremia, and mortality in patients with chronic kidney disease with and without congestive heart failure. 677–684; Waikar, S. S., G. C. Curhan, and S. M. Brunelli. 2011. Mortality associated with low serum sodium concentration in maintenance hemodialysis. *Am J Med* 124(1): 77–84.

120. Dong, J., et al. 2010. Low dietary sodium intake increases the death risk in peritoneal dialysis. *Clin J Am Soc Nephrol* 5(2): 240–247.

121. Zevallos, G., D. G. Oreopoulos, and M. L. Halperin. 2001. Hyponatremia in patients undergoing CAPD: role of water gain and/or malnutrition. *Perit Dial Int* 21(1): 72–76.

122. Johnson, R. J., et al. 2014. Hyperosmolarity drives hypertension and CKD—water and salt revisited. *Nat Rev Nephrol* 10(7): 415–420.

123. Nakayama. Dietary fructose causes tubulointerstitial injury in the normal rat kidney. F712–F720.

124. Johnson. Hyperosmolarity drives hypertension and CKD—water and salt revisited. 415–420.

125. Mulcahy, A., and V. Forbes. 2015. Intestinal failure and short bowel syndrome. *Medicine* 43(4): 239–243.

126. Barkas, F., et al. 2013. Electrolyte and acid-base disorders in inflammatory bowel disease. *Ann Gastroenterol* 26(1): 23–28; Schilli, R., et al. 1982. Comparison of the composition of faecal fluid in Crohn's disease and ulcerative colitis. *Gut* 23(4): 326–332; Vernia, P., et al. 1988.

Organic anions and the diarrhea of inflammatory bowel disease. *Dig Dis Sci* 33(11): 1353–1358; Beeken, W. L. 1975. Remediable defects in Crohn disease: a prospective study of 63 patients. *Arch Intern Med* 135(5): 686–690; Allan, R., et al. 1975. Changes in the bidirectional sodium flux across the intestinal mucosa in Crohn's disease. *Gut* 16(3): 201–204.

127. Delin. Factors regulating sodium balance in proctocolectomized patients with various ileal resections. 145–149.

128. Davidson, M. B., and A. I. Erlbaum. 1979. Role of ketogenesis in urinary sodium excretion: elucidation by nicotinic acid administration during fasting. *J Clin Endocrinol Metab* 49(6): 818–823.

129. Boulter, P. R., R. S. Hoffman, and R. A. Arky. Pattern of sodium excretion accompanying starvation. *Metabolism* 22(5): 675–683.

130. Bloom, W. L., and G. J. Azar. 1963. Similarities of carbohydrate deficiency and fasting. I. Weight loss, electrolyte excretion, and fatigue. 333–337.

131. Rabast, U., K. H. Vornberger, and M. Ehl. 1981. Loss of weight, sodium and water in obese persons consuming a high- or low-carbohydrate diet. *Ann Nutr Metab* 25(6): 341–349.

132. Krzywicki, H. J., et al. 1968. Metabolic aspects of acute starvation. *Am J Clin Nutr* 21(1): 87–97.

133. Runcie, J. 1971. Urinary sodium and potassium excretion in fasting obese subjects. *BMJ* 2(5752): 22–25.

134. Runcie, J., and T. E. Wheldon. 1976. Cyclic renal sodium excretion in women: evidence for a further control system mediating renal sodium loss [proceedings]. *J Physiol* 260(2): 59p.

135. Garnett, E. S., et al. 1968. The mobilization of osmotically inactive sodium during total starvation in man. *Clin Sci* 35(1): 93–103.

136. Ibid.

137. Simpson, F. O., et al. 1984. Iodide excretion in a salt-restriction trial. *N Z Med J* 97(770): 890–893.

138. Ibid.

139. Jantsch, J., et al. 2015. Cutaneous Na+ storage strengthens the antimicrobial barrier function of the skin and boosts macrophage-driven host defense. *Cell Metab* 21(3): 493–501.

140. Kaufman, A. M., G. Hellman, and R. G. Abramson. 1983. Renal salt wasting and metabolic acidosis with trimethoprim-sulfamethoxazole therapy. *Mt Sinai J Med* 50(3): 238–239.

141. Jantsch. Cutaneous Na+ storage strengthens the antimicrobial barrier function of the skin and boosts macrophage-driven host defense.

493–501; Wiig, H., et al. 2013. Immune cells control skin lymphatic electrolyte homeostasis and blood pressure. *J Clin Invest* 123(7): 2803–2815.

142. Woehrle, T., et al. 2010. Hypertonic stress regulates T cell function via pannexin-1 hemichannels and P2X receptors. *J Leukoc Biol* 88(6): 1181–1189.

143. http://www.ncbi.nlm.nih.gov/books/NBK50952/.

144. https://acmsf.food.gov.uk/sites/default/files/mnt/drupal_data/sources /files/multimedia/pdfs/acm740a.pdf.

145. Ibid.

146. McCarty, M. F., and J. J. DiNicolantonio. 2014. Bioavailable dietary phosphate, a mediator of cardiovascular disease, may be decreased with plant-based diets, phosphate binders, niacin, and avoidance of phosphate additives. *Nutrition* 30(7–8): 739–747.

147. Good, P. 2011. Do salt cravings in children with autistic disorders reveal low blood sodium depleting brain taurine and glutamine? *Med Hypotheses* 77(6): 1015–1021.

148. Ibid; http://rehydrate.org/resources/jianas.htm.

149. AlZahrani, Sinnert, and Gernsheimer. Acute kidney injury, sodium disorders, and hypercalcemia in the aging kidney: diagnostic and therapeutic management strategies in emergency medicine. 275–319.

150. Ibid; Luft. Clinical salt deficits. 559–563.

151. Urso, C., and G. Caimi. 2012. [Hyponatremic syndrome]. *Clin Ter* 163(1): e29–e39. [Article in Italian.]

152. Agarwal. Hyponatremic-hypertensive syndrome with renal ischemia: an underrecognized disorder. 1020–1024; Husain, M. K., et al. 1975. Nicotine-stimulated release of neurophysin and vasopressin in humans. *J Clin Endocrinol Metab* 41(06): 1113–1117.

CHAPTER 8: THE SALT FIX: GIVE YOUR BODY WHAT IT REALLY NEEDS

1. Wu, T., et al. 2002. Associations of serum C-reactive protein with fasting insulin, glucose, and glycosylated hemoglobin: the Third National Health and Nutrition Examination Survey, 1988–1994. *Am J Epidemiol* 155(1): 65–71; Palaniappan, L. P., M. R. Carnethon, and S. P. Fortmann. Heterogeneity in the relationship between ethnicity, BMI, and fasting insulin. *Diabetes Care* 25(8): 1351–1357; Lindeberg, S., et al. 1999. Low serum insulin in traditional Pacific Islanders—the Kitava Study. *Metabolism* 48(10): 1216–1219; Lindgarde, F., et al. 2004. Traditional versus agricultural lifestyle among Shuar women of

the Ecuadorian Amazon: effects on leptin levels. *Metabolism* 53(10): 1355–1358.

2. Reiser, S., et al. 1981. Serum insulin and glucose in hyperinsulinemic subjects fed three different levels of sucrose. *Am J Clin Nutr* 34(11): 2348–2358; Reiser, S., et al. 1979. Isocaloric exchange of dietary starch and sucrose in humans. II. Effect on fasting blood insulin, glucose, and glucagon and on insulin and glucose response to a sucrose load. *Am J Clin Nutr* 32(11): 2206–2216; Madero, M., et al. 2011. The effect of two energy-restricted diets, a low-fructose diet versus a moderate natural fructose diet, on weight loss and metabolic syndrome parameters: a randomized controlled trial. *Metabolism* 60(11): 1551–1559.

3. DiNicolantonio, J. J., J. H. O'Keefe, and S. C. Lucan, Added fructose: a principal driver of type 2 diabetes mellitus and its consequences. *Mayo Clin Proc* 90(3): 372–381.

4. Malaguarnera, M., et al. 2010. L-carnitine supplementation to diet: a new tool in treatment of nonalcoholic steatohepatitis—a randomized and controlled clinical trial. *Am J Gastroenterol* 105(6): 1338–1345; Zhang, J. J., et al. 2014. L-carnitine ameliorated fasting-induced fatigue, hunger, and metabolic abnormalities in patients with metabolic syndrome: a randomized controlled study. *Nutr J* 13: 110.

5. McCarty, M. F., and J. J. DiNicolantonio. 2014. The cardiometabolic benefits of glycine: is glycine an "antidote" to dietary fructose? *Open Heart* 1:e000103. doi:10.1136/openhrt-2014-000103.

6. http://www.pureencapsulations.com/media/Iodine.pdf.

7. Lucan, S. C., and J. J. DiNicolantonio. 2015. How calorie-focused thinking about obesity and related diseases may mislead and harm public health. An alternative. *Public Health Nutr* 18(4): 571–581.

8. Buu, L. M., and Y. C. Chen. 2014. Impact of glucose levels on expression of hypha-associated secreted aspartyl proteinases in *Candida albicans*. *J Biomed Sci* 21: 22; Vargas, S. L., et al. 1993. Modulating effect of dietary carbohydrate supplementation on *Candida albicans* colonization and invasion in a neutropenic mouse model. *Infect Immun* 61(2): 619–626; Vidotto, V., et al. 1996. Influence of fructose on *Candida albicans* germ tube production. *Mycopathologia* 135(2): 85–88; Brown, V., J. A. Sexton, and M. Johnston. 2006. A glucose sensor in *Candida albicans*. *Eukaryot Cell* 5(10): 1726–1737; Rodaki, A., et al. 2009. Glucose promotes stress resistance in the fungal pathogen *Candida albicans*. *Mol Biol Cell* 20(22): 4845–4855.

9. http://en.wikipedia.org/wiki/RealSalt; http://www.realsalt.com/wp-content/uploads/2013/03/realsalt_analysis.pdf; http://www.realsalt.com;

http://www.realsalt.com/sea-salt/comparing-real-salt-to-himalayan
-celtic/.

10. http://www.realsalt.com/sea-salt/know-your-salts/.

11. http://www.celticseasalt.com/about-us/faq/.

12. http://www.selinanaturally.com/makai-pure-deep-sea-salt/.

13. http://www.dowsers.com/Celtic Sea Salt Analysis.pdf; http://
healthfree.com/celtic_sea_salt.html.

14. http://themeadow.com/pages/minerals-in-himalayan-pink-salt
-spectral-analysis.

15. Ibid.

16. http://www.realsalt.com/sea-salt/know-your-salts/; http://drsircus.com
/medicine/salt/real-salt-celtic-salt-and-himalayan-salt - _edn1; http://
draxe.com/10-benefits-celtic-sea-salt-himalayan-salt/; http://www.louix
.org/the-difference-between-refined-salt-and-unrefined-salt/.

17. https://en.wikipedia.org/wiki/Kala_Namak.

18. http://seasonalitybylogovida.blogspot.com/2011/06/shock-value
-hawaiian-black-lava-sea.html.

19. http://www.sfsalt.com/black-hawaiian-sea-salt.

20. http://www.thespicehouse.com/spices/hawaiian-black-and-red-sea
-salt.

21. http://www.hawaiikaico.com/bulk.php.

22. http://themeadow.com/pages/about-hawaiian-sea-salt.

23. http://www.hawaiikaico.com/.

24. http://themeadow.com/pages/about-hawaiian-sea-salt.

25. http://k.b5z.net/i/u/2182313/f/Tech_Data_Sheet_-gourmet_salt
_-_black_hawaiian_lava_sea_salt-2.pdf; http://k.b5z.net/i/u/2182313/f
/Tech_Data_Sheet_-gourmet_salt_-_alaea_hawaiian_sea_salt-2.pdf.

26. http://www.realsalt.com/sea-salt/know-your-salts/.

27. http://articles.mercola.com/sites/articles/archive/2010/08/25/why
-has-this-lifesustaining-essential-nutrient-been-vilified-by-doctors
.aspx; http://articles.mercola.com/sites/articles/archive/2011/09/20/salt
-myth.aspx.

28. http://www.smh.com.au/national/sushi-linked-to-thyroid-illness
-20110730-1i5ul.html.

29. Payne, C. L., et al. 2016. Are edible insects more or less 'healthy' than
commonly consumed meats? A comparison using two nutrient profiling models developed to combat over- and undernutrition. *Eur J Clin
Nutr* 70(3): 285–291.

30. Bacchi, E., et al. 2012. Metabolic effects of aerobic training and resistance training in type 2 diabetic subjects: a randomized controlled trial (the RAED2 study). *Diabetes Care* 35(4): 676–682.

31. Hansen, E., et al. 2012. Insulin sensitivity after maximal and endurance resistance training. *J Strength Cond Res* 26(2): 327–334.

APPENDIX I

1. Graudal, N. 2005. Commentary: possible role of salt intake in the development of essential hypertension. *Int J Epidemiol* 34: 972–974.

2. Ibid.

3. Ibid.

4. Chapman, C. B., and T. B. Gibbons. 1950. The diet and hypertension: a review. *Medicine (Baltimore)* 29(1): 29–69.

5. Ibid.

6. Ibid.

7. Ibid.

8. Ibid.

9. Grollman, A. R., et al. 1945. Sodium restriction in the diet for hypertension. *JAMA* 129(8): 533–537.

10. Dahl, L. K., and R. A. Love. 1954. Evidence for relationship between sodium (chloride) intake and human essential hypertension. *AMA Arch Intern Med* 94(4): 525–531; Meneely, G. R., R. G. Tucker, and W. J. Darby. 1952. Chronic sodium chloride toxicity in the albino rat. I. Growth on a purified diet containing various levels of sodium chloride. *J Nutr* 48(4): 489–498.

11. http://www.forbes.com/sites/realspin/2015/04/09/if-you-must-have-a-dietary-culprit-at-least-pick-the-right-one/.

12. Dahl, L. K. 2005. Possible role of salt intake in the development of essential hypertension. 1960. *Int J Epidemiol* 34(5): 967–972; discussion 972–974, 975–978.

13. Keys, A. 1953. Atherosclerosis: a problem in newer public health. *J Mt Sinai Hosp N Y* 20(2): 118–139.

14. Dietary fat and its relation to heart attacks and strokes. Report by the Central Committee for Medical and Community Program of the American Heart Association. *JAMA* 175(5): 389–391.

15. Hall, C. E., and O. Hall. 1966. Salt hypertension induced by drinking saline and the effect of different concentrations of sucrose and maltose upon its development. *Tex Rep Biol Med* 24(3): 445–456; Hall, C. E., and O. Hall. 1966. Comparative effectiveness of glucose and

sucrose in enhancement of hypersalimentation and salt hypertension. *Proc Soc Exp Biol Med* 123(2): 370–374.

16. Brunner, H. R., et al. 1972. Essential hypertension: renin and aldosterone, heart attack and stroke. *N Engl J Med* 286(9): 441–449.

17. Ahrens, R. A. 1974. Sucrose, hypertension, and heart disease: an historical perspective. *Am J Clin Nutr* 27(4): 403–422.

18. Harper, A. E. 1978. Dietary goals—a skeptical view. *Am J Clin Nutr* 31(2): 310–321.

19. Walker, A. R. 1975. Sucrose, hypertension, and heart disease. *Am J Clin Nutr* 28(3): 195–200.

20. Meneely, G. R., and H. D. Battarbee. 1976. High sodium-low potassium environment and hypertension. *Am J Cardiol* 38(6): 768–785; Freis, E. D. 1976. Salt, volume and the prevention of hypertension. *Circulation* 53(4): 589–595.

21. http://zerodisease.com/archive/Dietary_Goals_For_The_United _States.pdf.

22. Harper. Dietary goals—a skeptical view. 310–321.

23. Simpson, F. O. 1979. Salt and hypertension: a sceptical review of the evidence. *Clin Sci (Lond)* 57(Suppl 5): 463s–480s.

24. Swales, J. D. 1980. Dietary salt and hypertension. *Lancet* 1(8179): 1177–1179.

25. Preuss, M. B., and H. G. Preuss. 1980. The effects of sucrose and sodium on blood pressures in various substrains of Wistar rats. *Lab Invest* 43(2): 101–107.

26. Yamori, Y., et al. 1981. Hypertension and diet: multiple regression analysis in a Japanese farming community. *Lancet* 1(8231): 1204–1205.

27. http://content.time.com/time/covers/0,16641,19820315,00.html.

28. Rebello, T., R. E. Hodges, and J. L. Smith. 1983. Short-term effects of various sugars on antinatriuresis and blood pressure changes in normotensive young men. *Am J Clin Nutr* 38(1): 84–94.

29. Hodges, R. E., and T. Rebello. 1983. Carbohydrates and blood pressure. *Ann Intern Med* 98(5 Pt 2): 838–841.

30. Boon, N. A., and J. K. Aronson. 1985. Dietary salt and hypertension: treatment and prevention. *BMJ (Clin Res Ed)* 290(6473): 949–950.

31. Intersalt: an international study of electrolyte excretion and blood pressure. Results for 24 hour urinary sodium and potassium excretion. Intersalt Cooperative Research Group. *BMJ.* 1988. 297(6644): 319–328.

32. Dustan, H. P., and K. A. Kirk. 1989. Corcoran lecture: the case for or against salt in hypertension. Arthur Curtis Corcoran, MD (1909–1965). Tribute and prelude to Corcoran Lecture of 1988. *Hypertension* 13(6 Pt 2): 696–705.

33. Law, M. R., C. D. Frost, and N. J. Wald. 1991. By how much does dietary salt reduction lower blood pressure? III—Analysis of data from trials of salt reduction. *BMJ* 302(6780): 819–824.

34. The fifth report of the Joint National Committee on Detection, Evaluation, and Treatment of High Blood Pressure (JNC V). *Arch Intern Med.* 1993. 153(2): 154–183.

35. Alderman, M. H., et al. 1995. Low urinary sodium is associated with greater risk of myocardial infarction among treated hypertensive men. *Hypertension* 25(6): 1144–1152.

36. Graudal, N. A., A. M. Galloe, and P. Garred. 1998. Effects of sodium restriction on blood pressure, renin, aldosterone, catecholamines, cholesterols, and triglyceride: a meta-analysis. *JAMA* 279(17): 1383–1391.

37. Sacks, F. M., et al. 2001. Effects on blood pressure of reduced dietary sodium and the Dietary Approaches to Stop Hypertension (DASH) diet. DASH-Sodium Collaborative Research Group. *N Engl J Med* 344(1): 3–10.

38. Vollmer, W. M., et al. 2001. Effects of diet and sodium intake on blood pressure: subgroup analysis of the DASH-sodium trial. *Ann Intern Med* 135(12): 1019–1028.

39. Harsha, D. W., et al. 2004. Effect of dietary sodium intake on blood lipids: results from the DASH-sodium trial. *Hypertension* 43(2): 393–398.

40. Raben, A., et al. 2002. Sucrose compared with artificial sweeteners: different effects on ad libitum food intake and body weight after 10 wk of supplementation in overweight subjects. *Am J Clin Nutr* 76(4): 721–729.

41. Brown, C. M., et al. 2008. Fructose ingestion acutely elevates blood pressure in healthy young humans. *Am J Physiol Regul Integr Comp Physiol* 294(3): R730–R737.

42. Perez-Pozo, S. E., et al. 2010. Excessive fructose intake induces the features of metabolic syndrome in healthy adult men: role of uric acid in the hypertensive response. *Int J Obes (Lond)* 34(3): 454–461.

43. Stolarz-Skrzypek, K., et al. 2011. Fatal and nonfatal outcomes, incidence of hypertension, and blood pressure changes in relation to urinary sodium excretion. *JAMA* 305(17): 1777–1785.

44. Malik, A. H., et al. 2014. Impact of sugar-sweetened beverages on blood pressure. *Am J Cardiol* 113(9): 1574–1580.

45. Te Morenga, L. A., et al. 2014. Dietary sugars and cardiometabolic risk: systematic review and meta-analyses of randomized controlled trials of the effects on blood pressure and lipids. *Am J Clin Nutr* 100(1): 65–79.

46. Adler, A. J., et al. 2014. Reduced dietary salt for the prevention of cardiovascular disease. *Cochrane Database Syst Rev* (12): Cd009217.

47. Graudal, N., et al. 2014. Compared with usual sodium intake, low- and excessive-sodium diets are associated with increased mortality: a meta-analysis. *Am J Hypertens* 27(9): 1129–1137.

48. http://health.gov/dietaryguidelines/2015-scientific-report/pdfs/scientific-report-of-the-2015-dietary-guidelines-advisory-committee.pdf.

49. Mente, A., et al. 2016. Associations of urinary sodium excretion with cardiovascular events in individuals with and without hypertension: a pooled analysis of data from four studies. *Lancet* 388(10043): 465–475.

50. Kelly, J., et al. 2016. The effect of dietary sodium modification on blood pressure in adults with systolic blood pressure less than 140 mmHg: a systematic review. *JBI Database System Rev Implement Rep* 14(6): 196–237.

51. http://zerodisease.com/archive/Dietary_Goals_For_The_United_States.pdf.

52. https://thescienceofnutrition.files.wordpress.com/2014/03/dietary-goals-for-the-united-states.pdf.

53. http://www.health.gov/dietaryguidelines/1980thin.pdf.

54. http://www.health.gov/dietaryguidelines/1985thin.pdf.

55. http://www.health.gov/dietaryguidelines/1990thin.pdf.

56. http://www.cnpp.usda.gov/sites/default/files/dietary_guidelines_for_americans/1995DGConsumerBrochure.pdf.

57. http://www.health.gov/dietaryguidelines/dga2000/dietgd.pdf.

58. http://www.nal.usda.gov/fnic/DRI/DRI_Energy/energy_full_report.pdf.

59. http://www.health.gov/dietaryguidelines/dga2005/document/pdf/dga2005.pdf.

60. http://www.health.gov/dietaryguidelines/dga2010/dietaryguidelines2010.pdf.

61. http://health.gov/dietaryguidelines/2015-scientific-report/pdfs/scientific-report-of-the-2015-dietary-guidelines-advisory-committee.pdf.

62. http://zerodisease.com/archive/Dietary_Goals_For_The_United _States.pdf.

63. https://thescienceofnutrition.files.wordpress.com/2014/03/dietary -goals-for-the-united-states.pdf.

64. http://www.health.gov/dietaryguidelines/1980thin.pdf.

65. http://www.health.gov/dietaryguidelines/1985thin.pdf.

66. http://www.health.gov/dietaryguidelines/1990thin.pdf.

67. http://www.cnpp.usda.gov/sites/default/files/dietary_guidelines_for _americans/1995DGConsumerBrochure.pdf.

68. http://www.health.gov/dietaryguidelines/dga2000/dietgd.pdf.

69. Trumbo, P., et al. 2002. Dietary reference intakes for energy, carbohy-drate, fiber, fat, fatty acids, cholesterol, protein and amino acids. *J Am Diet Assoc* 102(11): 1621–1630.

70. http://www.health.gov/dietaryguidelines/dga2005/document/pdf /dga2005.pdf.

71. http://www.health.gov/dietaryguidelines/dga2010/dietaryguidelines 2010.pdf.

72. http://health.gov/dietaryguidelines/2015-scientific-report/pdfs /scientific-report-of-the-2015-dietary-guidelines-advisory-committee .pdf.

APPENDIX 2

1. Luft, F. C. 2015. Clinical salt deficits. *Pflugers Arch* 467(3): 559–563; Shihab, F. S., et al. 1997. Sodium depletion enhances fibrosis and the expression of TGF-beta1 and matrix proteins in experimental chronic cyclosporine nephropathy. *Am J Kidney Dis* 30(1): 71–81.

2. Saleh, M. 2014. Sepsis-associated renal salt wasting: how much is too much? *BMJ Case Rep.* doi:10.1136/bcr-2013-201838.

3. AlZahrani, A., R. Sinnert, and J. Gernsheimer. 2013. Acute kidney injury, sodium disorders, and hypercalcemia in the aging kidney: di-agnostic and therapeutic management strategies in emergency medi-cine. *Clin Geriatr Med* 29(1): 275–319; Vroman, R. 2011. Electrolyte imbalances. Part 1: Sodium balance disorders. *EMS World* 40(2): 37–38, 40–43; Khow, K. S., and T. Y. Yong. 2014. Hyponatraemia associ-ated with trimethoprim use. *Curr Drug Saf* 9(1): 79–82.

ACKNOWLEDGMENTS

. . . .

To my wife, Megan, you have always believed in me and have been my biggest supporter. You were there every step of the way and without you this book would not have happened. I love you with all of my heart and I am so grateful to have you as my wife. To my amazing children, AJ and Emma, you two bring me so much joy. Thank you for being my cheering section and reminding me to appreciate the little things in life. I will never forget your two tiny faces beaming with pride as you yelled, "Congratulations!" for finishing my "workbook." I love you both so much.

My deepest thanks and gratitude to all of those involved who have helped to make this book become a reality.

To my agent, Bonnie Solow, your belief in me is the reason why this book is possible. I can't thank you enough for your expertise and support.

To Mariska van Aalst, thank you for bringing my research to life. This book would not be what it is without your work.

To Donna Loffredo, Heather Jackson, Diana Baroni, Rebecca Marsh, Stephanie Davis, and the entire team at Harmony Books, Crown Publishing Group, and Penguin Random House for believing in this project and bringing it to fruition. I cannot thank you enough.

To my friend David Harris, thank you so much for your personal anecdote and for always making me laugh.

To my colleagues Jose Carlos Souto, Sean Lucan, Dmitri Vasin, and

David Unwin, who contributed by humanizing my research through personal anecdotes. Thank you.

To my colleagues Dr. James O'Keefe and Dr. Chip Lavie, you have provided guidance and support over the years for which I will be forever grateful.

To my cousin and friend Ryan DiMillo, for spearheading website development and digital marketing, and keeping me laughing along the way.

To my mom and dad, thank you for your constant support and making me the person I am today. I am so grateful to have you as my parents.

To my family and friends, I could not have done this without your unwavering love and support. Thank you so much.

INDEX

· · · · · · · · · · · · ·

and sodium, 98, 143, 155
sugar as cause of, 60, 64, 76, 145
diastolic blood pressure, 8, 52–53, 141
Dietary Approaches to Stop
    Hypertension (DASH)-Sodium
    trial, 56, 87, 192
Dietary Goals (1977), 44–46, 59, 64,
    190, 194, 195
Dietary Guidelines (1980), 64, 194, 195
Dietary Guidelines (2005), 56, 194, 195
Dietary Guidelines (2010), 65, 194, 195
Dietary Guidelines for Americans
    (1995), 55, 57, 194, 195
Dietary Guidelines for Americans
    (2015), 58, 195
Dinesen, Isak, 1
disease, 32–34, 42, 61–64, 119, 129, 158,
    186
    See also specific diseases
diuretics, 12, 47, 97, 98, 162
docosahexaenoic acid (DHA), 21, 23
dopamine, 113–15, 120, 166
dressings, 172, 198
drugs, 106–10, 112–15, 120, 196
    See also medication; specific drugs
Dustan, Harriet P., 191

edema, 154
electrolytes, 15–18, 26, 128
elephants, 29–30
Elliot, Paul, 54, 55
endurance resistance training, 182
energy, 92, 93, 100, 142–43, 181–84
essential hypertension, 77, 84
Europe, 33–34, 62
    See also specific countries
euvolemic hyponatremia, 157
excretion
    by kidneys, 17, 19, 48, 72–73, 105, 146
    of salt, 18, 96, 121, 122, 124, 125, 151,
        154, 168
    in urine, 26, 125, 126
exercise, 120, 130–37, 181–84
Ezekiel bread, 166–67, 170

fasting, 95, 120, 151, 152
fat, 2, 58, 91–95, 98–99, 116, 182, 184

    See also saturated fat
fatigue, 142, 143
fatty liver, 96, 144, 160, 169
fish, 17–18, 20, 172
flavor, 172
Folkow, Bjorn, 43, 55, 74
food, 22, 170–73, 179, 187, 188, 197–98
    See also specific foods
food poisoning, 155–56
France, 33, 66, 171
Friedrich-Alexander-University
    Erlangen-Nuremberg (Ger.), 119
fructose, 99, 112, 116, 144, 149, 164–65
fruit, 36, 113, 163, 166, 171, 172

garlic salt, 134, 180, 183
Garnett, E. S., 152
gastrointestinal disorders, 129
gastrointestinal system, 173
ghrelin, 165
Giampietro, Ottavio, 76
glucocorticoids, 80
glucose, 91, 94–96, 99, 100, 143–44, 149,
    164–66, 181–82, 184
glucose challenge test, 161
glycine, 169
goiter, 131, 132, 154, 178
Good Calories, Bad Calories (Taubes),
    90
gorillas, 30
Gower, John, 112
Graudal, Niels, 192, 193
Guyton, Arthur, 48

habituation, 104
Harper, A. E., 190
Harris, David, 133
Hawaiian black lava salt, 177–78
Hawaiian red Alaea salt, 177–78
Hawaii Kai Corporation, 177–78
headache, 4, 5
health, 72, 99
Heaney, Robert, 70
heart attack, 9, 28, 50, 57, 64, 67
heart disease
    causes of, 51, 64–89, 190
    and salt, 10, 31–32, 34, 68, 86, 89

ABOUT THE AUTHOR

James DiNicolantonio, PharmD, is a cardiovascular research scientist and doctor of pharmacy at Saint Luke's Mid America Heart Institute in Kansas City, Missouri. A well-respected and internationally known scientist and expert on health and nutrition, he has contributed extensively to health policy. He has published over two hundred scientific papers in the medical literature. Dr. DiNicolantonio has testified in front of the Canadian Senate on the drivers of obesity and the harmful effects that refined carbohydrates and sugar have on our health. He has published numerous high-profile articles on nutrition in the lay press, including the *New York Times*, *Forbes*, and *U.S. News & World Report*. He serves as the associate editor of *BMJ Open Heart*, a journal published in partnership with the British Cardiovascular Society. He is also on the editorial advisory board of several other medical journals, including *Progress in Cardiovascular Diseases*, *Journal of Insulin Resistance*, and *International Journal of Clinical Pharmacology and Toxicology*. He lives in Fairport, New York.